SELF-ASSESSMENT FOR
MRCP (PART 1)

D0243002

ıte

ıc

Self-Assessment for MRCP (Part 1) Paediatrics

Fiona O. Finlay
BSc DGM DRCOG DCH MRCGP MRCP

Jonathan O'B. Hourihane
MB BCh BAO MRCPI

Both of the Child Health Department
Southampton General Hospital
Southampton

Blackwell
Science

This book is dedicated to Simon and Yvonne

© 1995 by
Blackwell Science Ltd
Editorial Offices:
Osney Mead, Oxford OX2 0EL
25 John Street, London WC1N 2BL
23 Ainslie Place, Edinburgh EH3 6AJ
238 Main Street, Cambridge
Massachusetts 02142, USA
54 University Street, Carlton
Victoria 3053, Australia

Other Editorial Offices:
Arnette Blackwell SA
1, rue de Lille, 75007 Paris
France

Blackwell Wissenschafts-Verlag GmbH
Kurfürstendamm 57
10707 Berlin, Germany

Feldgasse 13, A-1238 Wien
Austria

First published 1995

Set by Semantic Graphics, Singapore
Printed and bound in Great Britain by
Hartnolls Ltd, Bodmin, Cornwall

DISTRIBUTORS

Marston Book Services Ltd
PO Box 87
Oxford OX2 0DT
(*Orders*: Tel: 01865 791155
        Fax: 01865 791927
        Telex: 837515)

North America
Blackwell Science, Inc.
238 Main Street
Cambridge, MA 02142
(*Orders*: Tel: 800 215-1000
        617 876-7000
        Fax: 617 492-5263)

Australia
Blackwell Science Pty Ltd
54 University Street
Carlton, Victoria 3053
(*Orders*: Tel: 03 347-0300
        Fax: 03 349-3016)

A catalogue record for this title
is available from the British Library

ISBN 0-86542-955-3

Contents

Introduction

The advent of MRCP Paediatrics Part 1 in 1993 was a major step forward for paediatricians in training. The 'adult' MRCP Part 1 was often a stumbling block as little of the syllabus and few of the questions addressed issues and problems of child health and paediatrics. The current format of MRCP Paeds Part 1 still retains questions on adult medicine but these are asked in ways that are more general and more easily addressed by paediatricians. It is possible that, when the proposed British College of Paediatricians is established, it will institute a purely paediatric examination, similar to those of the Colleges of Surgeons, Anaesthetists, and Obstetricians and Gynaecologists.

The multiple choice question (MCQ) is well established in medical education. It would be an exception to qualify from medical school without gaining some proficiency in the necessary techniques required for survival. Negative marking demands a disciplined approach to the paper, requiring the candidate to recognise things that he or she does not know. Each question has a root phrase or statement and five related stems. Each stem is a separate statement that must be evaluated solely on its own merits. Just because stems A and B are true does not mean that stem C is false.

This self-assessment book hopefully reflects the (unpublished) syllabus for the MRCP Paeds Part 1 and the needs of paediatricians in training who are sitting it. The proportion of questions in MRCP Part 1 that are related to basic sciences has increased since the examination was introduced. We have entitled one of the chapters 'Basic *and* Clinical Sciences' to reflect some of the topics a candidate needs to cover in his or her studies. Some questions relate to fundamentals of medical practice such as heart sounds or applied anatomy — these are popular topics for MCQs as the basic facts and findings rarely change. Neither author claims to be a scientist and some readers may need to look elsewhere for questions regarding cellular and molecular biology. There is certainly a need for such a book.

The questions (more than 300) are entirely new. It is worth noting that topics in journals and reviews are not necessarily dogma and we have deliberately avoided basing questions on areas of controversy.

The answers to the questions in this book act as a primary source of information (especially if the condition is completely unknown to the candidate!). All the answers should be easily available in one of the major textbooks listed in the bibliography. We feel anyone under-taking postgraduate study and examinations should possess a personal copy of a major text to allow for wider reading around a particular topic or area of interest.

The book is divided into sections relating to body systems and related disciplines of paediatrics. The final section of the book is of sixty questions laid out in an examination format. We would strongly recommend that candidates try to 'sit' this section under examination conditions, giving themselves 2¼ hours to complete the paper. It is difficult, but worthwhile, to avoid looking at the answers as one goes along.

Good luck.

1: Basic and Clinical Sciences

Answers to this section are to be found
between pages 8 and 17

QUESTIONS

BS1 In DNA analysis

A Large DNA fragments migrate faster than small ones during electrophoresis

B Recombinant vector plasmids are amplified in *Escherichia coli*

C The technique of Southern blotting is used to transfer single strands of DNA onto a nitrocellulose filter or nylon membrane

D Restriction fragment length polymorphisms can be used as markers for genetic disorders if close to the gene of interest

E Storing DNA is difficult due to its instability

BS2 Cerebral blood flow

A Accounts for 15% of cardiac output at rest

B Is increased by a rise in concentration of CO_2

C Is constant for regions of the brain, irrespective of ongoing cerebral activity

D Is altered by damage to the sympathetic chain

E Increases in response to cerebral oedema

BS3 Hypercapnia is associated with

A Papilloedema

B Reduced intracranial pressure

C Increased blood pH

D Perioral paraesthesiae

E Depression of the respiratory centre

BS4 The ulna

A Is the lateral bone of the forearm in the anatomical position

B Is shorter than the radius

C Has a distal end which is larger than the proximal end

D Fits around the humerus via the semilunar notch

E Has an insertion point for the brachialis muscle

1

BS5 The following statements regarding thyroxine binding globulin (TBG) are correct

A Ten per cent of T4 is bound to TBG

B Levels of TBG are increased in newborn infants

C TBG levels may be deficient as a result of an X-linked dominant disorder

D TBG is synthesised in the liver

E TBG deficiency may not be detectable on Guthrie testing

BS6 In the skin

A The mature epidermis is constantly renewed by meiotic division of cells in the basal layer

B The total lifespan of the epidermal cell is approximately 60 days

C The Langerhans cells contain melanosomes

D Hair follicles regenerate if destroyed

E Apocrine glands remain dormant until puberty

BS7 Natural killer cells

A Recognise free virus particles

B Kill cells by apoptosis

C Are activated by interferons

D Are derived from eosinophils

E Kill cells more effectively if the cells are coated in antibody

BS8 The Krebs' cycle

A Is also known as the citric acid cycle

B Occurs in the cytosol

C Involves the formation of one high energy bond each cycle

D Starts with the conversation of succinate to fumarate

E Operates in anaerobic conditions

BS9 In mitotic cellular division

A Cells are in anaphase before division

B Prophase is the first phase of mitosis

C At telophase the chromatids have reached opposite poles of the cell

D In metaphase the paired chromatids are lined up along the equatorial plane of the cell

E At interphase each chromatid passes to one or other daughter cell

BS10 Cardiac muscle
A Responds in an 'all or nothing' fashion to electrical stimulation
B Has different refractory periods in the atria and the ventricles
C Is a type of smooth muscle
D Decreases its contraction time when the heart rate increases
E Conducts action potentials more quickly than skeletal muscle

BS11 Myoglobin
A Facilitates the movement of oxygen within muscle
B Consists of a double polypeptide chain
C Largely assumes an alpha-helical conformation
D Has a lower affinity for oxygen than haemoglobin
E Has a hyperbolic shaped dissociation curve

BS12 Regarding renal function
A The normal glomerular basement membrane does not filter inulin from plasma
B Blood flow through the kidney is proportional to tissue mass
C Creatinine clearance overestimates glomerular filtration rate (GFR) in patients with renal impairment
D Dehydration may cause overestimation of creatinine levels
E Creatinine levels are maintained until GFR falls below 70%

BS13 The following statements regarding water are correct
A Expiration from the lungs and skin accounts for 40–50% of fluid output
B The water content of an infant is 40–45%
C The water soluble vitamins are A, D, E, K
D The ascending loop of Henle is impermeable to water
E The average insensible water loss in an infant is 1 g/kg/h

BS14 The umbilical artery
A Is a branch of the external iliac artery
B Persists postnatally as the ligamentum teres
C Is single in 1% of cases
D Carries oxygenated blood to the fetus
E Lies cephalad to the vein on a cross section of the cord

BS15 With regard to gene structure and function
A DNA exists as a triple stranded helix
B In DNA the pyrimidine bases are cytosine and uracil
C In RNA uracil replaces thymine
D DNA probes are produced using reverse transcriptase
E Coding sequences are termed introns

BS16 The following are examples of type 3 hypersensitivity reactions
A Post-streptococcal glomerulonephritis
B BCG immunisation
C House dust mite sensitive asthma
D Autoimmune haemolytic anaemia
E Farmer's lung

BS17 Regarding the cranial nerves
A The fourth cranial nerve is the abducent nerve
B The chorda tympani carries fibres of the seventh nerve
C A seventh nerve palsy causes fasciculation of the tongue
D Bilateral seventh nerve palsies are a feature of Lyme disease
E The oculomotor nerve supplies the lateral rectus muscles

BS18 With regard to lung development
A Alveoli begin to appear at 20 weeks gestation
B The respiratory bud develops from the foregut
C Type 1 pneumocytes are associated with surfactant production and excretion
D Oligohydramnios is associated with lung hypoplasia
E Glucocorticoids influence the maturation of lung connective tissue

BS19 Antidiuretic hormone (ADH) release is stimulated by
A Hypotension
B Excess water intake
C Angiotension
D Nicotine
E Alcohol

BS20 With regard to complement
A C2 is the most abundant form of complement
B Complement activation facilitates phagocytosis
C C-reactive protein (CRP) fixes complement
D The complement system directly causes a burst in respiratory activity of neutrophils
E Mast cell degranulation is dependent on the presence of bacterial lipopolysaccharide

BS21 With regard to heart sounds
A The first sound is loud in the presence of anaemia
B There is fixed splitting of the second heart sound in the presence of an atrial septal defect
C There is paradoxical splitting of the second heart sound in aortic stenosis
D The first heart sound is quiet in mitral stenosis
E The fourth sound occurs just after the first sound

BS22 Insulin
A Increases the rate of fatty acid synthesis
B Inhibits glycolysis
C Consists of four peptide chains
D Is formed from pre-insulin in the Golgi apparatus
E Decreases gluconeogenesis

BS23 Thyroxine (T4) excess
A Causes enzyme induction
B Decreases Na/K$^+$ ATPase activity
C Decreases serum cholesterol
D Causes a widening of pulse pressure
E Causes positive feedback on the hypothalmic–pituitary axis

BS24 Simple columnar epithelium is found in the following sites
A The stomach
B The upper oesophagus
C The sweat glands
D The uterus
E The loop of Henle

BS25 With regard to renal tract development
A The kidney derives from the metanephros
B The fetal kidney has a lobulated appearance
C The renal pelvis forms from the ureteric bud
D The urinary bladder is formed from the cloaca
E New nephrons continue to form until term

BS26 The alternative pathway of complement activation
A Involves linkage of bound antibody to C1q
B Causes breakdown of C3 to C3a and C3b
C Is activated by microbial lipopolysaccharide
D May cause release of anaphylatoxins
E Generates the C3 splitting enzyme known as C4b2b

BS27 The following statements are correct considering chromosomes
A Mitosis is the nuclear division giving rise to the gametes
B In the basic haploid set, $n = 2$
C Trisomy 21 is an example of a polyploid state
D A chimera is the presence of two different cell lines derived from one zygote
E Angelman's syndrome shows uniparental disomy

BS28 With regard to the mechanism of breathing
A The alveolar ventilation = (tidal volume – dead space) × respiratory rate
B The physiological dead space is about half of the tidal volume
C During each breath the volume of gas taken in or given out equals the tidal volume
D The volume expired from maximum inspiration to maximum expiration is the total lung capacity
E The volume remaining in the lung after maximum expiration is the functional residual capacity

BS29 Colostrum
A Production starts on the first postnatal day
B Is replaced by mature breast milk by three days
C Production is usually 150 ml/day

D Has higher casein levels than mature breast milk
E Has less fat than mature human milk

BS30 Synaptic transmission
A Only occurs in a forward direction
B Can be fatigued by repetitive stimulation
C Is decreased by a rise of pH
D May increase after repetitive stimulation
E May be blocked by strychnine

ANSWERS

BS1

A False — small fragments migrate faster

B True

C True

D True — the 'lod' score is an index of proximity

E False — once extracted, DNA is stable and can be stored indefinitely, so samples taken from affected individuals can be saved for future study of other family members

BS2

A True

B True — the association of CO_2 with water releases hydrogen ions. This increased acidosis causes local vasodilatation and hence increased cerebral blood flow. It is possible that this local response to increased acidosis causes increased removal of the hydrogen ions and hence correction of the abnormality and maintenance of homoeostais

C False — localised changes of flow can be seen when various tasks are undertaken such as reading (increased occipital flow) or squeezing a tennis ball (increased flow to the motor cortex)

D False — autonomic control is of little importance in cerebral blood flow which responds more to changes of pH and blood pressure

E False — cerebral oedema may cause loss of the autoregulation of cerebral blood flow which may fall to critical levels. Direct measurement of intracranial pressure and systemic blood pressure may allow calculation of cerebral blood flow and permit its maintenance between values of approximately 50 and 70 ml/g brain tissue/min

BS3

A True

B False — intracranial pressure is increased due to cerebral vasodilatation

C False — blood pH is reduced as is urinary pH

D False — paraesthesiae are associated with hyperventilation and therefore with a decreased CO_2

E True — a high partial pressure of CO_2 depresses the respiratory centre in the reticular formation in the medulla

BS4

A False — it is the medial bone
B False — it is longer than the radius
C False — the distal end is small and round and has a blunt projection on its posterior side (the styloid process)
D True — the deep semilunar notch fits around the trochlea of the humerus
E True — a roughened area called the tuberosity is the insertion point for the brachialis muscle

BS5

A False — TBG binds about 75% of T4 and 70% of T3
B True — levels are also increased in pregnancy and with the administration of oestrogens
C True — there is also a harmless X-linked dominant anomaly which causes an elevated TBG
D True — it is a glycoprotein
E True — Guthrie testing assays TSH levels

BS6

A False — only germ cells divide by meiosis
B False — skin turnover is usually 20–30 days
C False — Birbeck granules are a characteristic of these cells that are probably derived from bone marrow
D False — scars are always devoid of hair and other adenexae such as sweat glands and nerve endings
E True — apocrine glands are located in the axillae, groin and perineum

BS7

A False — natural killer cells recognise cells that have been infected by viruses
B True — this method of cellular destruction is characterised by nuclear fragmentation rather than cell lysis secondary to membrane disruption

C True — interferons are released by virally infected cells and act as a signal to attract natural killer cells

D False — natural killer cells are lymphocytes. Eosinophils are a separate cell line but are also involved in extracellular killing, particularly of parasites

E True — antibody binding brings the natural killer cell very close to the infected cell to allow extracellular killing

BS8

A True — it is also known as the tricarboxylic acid cycle

B False — the reactions of the Krebs' cycle occur within mitochondria, glycolysis occurs in the cytosol

C True

D False — most fuels enter the Krebs' cycle as the two carbon molecule acetyl CoA which binds with the four carbon molecule oxaloacetate

E False — the Krebs' cycle requires a supply of NAD^+ and FAD and operates only in aerobic conditions

BS9

A False — cells are in interphase before cell division

B True

C True

D True

E False — this stage is known as anaphase

BS10

A True — this is similar to nerve fibres. It is due to the nature of intercellular connections of the myofibrils which offer very low resistance to the passage of electrical signals

B True — the atrial refractory period is 0.15 s and the ventricular refractory period is 0.3 s. This can be seen on an ECG that shows complete heart block when intrinsic atrial activity causes the p waves to be more frequent than the QRS complexes of intrinsic ventricular activity

C False — cardiac muscle is striated and is more like skeletal muscle

D False — in response to faster rates the cardiac muscle's refractory time decreases

E False — cardiac muscle conducts at 0.3–0.5 m/s, about 10 times more slowly than skeletal muscle and 250 times more slowly than large nerve fibres. The specialised electrical conducting fibres in the heart can conduct up to 4 m/s

BS11

A True

B False — it is a single polypeptide chain of 153 residues

C True

D False — myoglobin has a higher affinity for oxygen than haemoglobin. Therefore oxygen passes from haemoglobin in the blood to myoglobin in the muscle

E True — haemoglobin has a sigmoidal shaped dissociation curve and therefore dissociates from oxygen more completely

BS12

A False — inulin is almost completely filtered and is used experimentally to measure glomerular filtration rate

B False — the cortex has a larger blood flow per unit mass than the medulla

C True — this is due to a larger proportion of urinary creatinine originating from tubular excretion rather than glomerular filtration

D False — unlike urea levels, creatinine levels are not influenced greatly by dehydration

E True

BS13

A False — insensible losses account for about 10% of output

B False — the water content of an infant is 70–75%

C False — these are the fat soluble vitamins

D False — about 65% of glomerular filtrate is reabsorbed in the proximal tubule

E True

BS14

A False — it is a branch of the internal iliac artery. When catheterised for arterial blood sampling in neonates it can be differentiated on X-ray from a catheterised umbilical vein by the initial downward loop of the catheter to enter the internal iliac artery

B False — the bilateral umbilical arteries persist as the lateral umbilical ligaments. The ligamentum teres is the vestige of the umbilical vein

C True — the presence of a single umbilical artery is associated in approximately 40% of cases with a variety of anomalies, particularly of the renal tract, which may prompt early renal investigations

D False — *in utero* the artery carries deoxygenated blood from the fetus to the placenta

E False — the usually paired umbilical arteries lie caudal to the umbilical vein. The arteries are muscular and stand out from the cut surface of the cord. The more patulous vein whose wall is less muscular lies more flush and bleeds more easily

BS15

A False — it exists as a double stranded helix with the order of bases on one strand complementary to those of the other strand

B False — pyrimidine bases are cytosine and thymine, purine bases are adenine and guanine

C True — ribose replaces deoxyribose as the sugar moiety

D True

E False — the coding sequences of genes are called exons and the intervening sequences introns. Greater than 90% of the genome consists of non-coding DNA. The function of this non-coding DNA is not yet clearly defined

BS16

A True — type 3 hypersensitivity is mediated by immune complex deposition. Nephrotic syndrome after quartan malaria is another type 3 reaction

B False

C False — house dust mite sensitive asthma is an example of IgE-mediated atopy or anaphylactic, type 1 hypersensitivity

D False — this is typical type 2 cytotoxic antibody dependent hypersensitivity. Cells, in this case red blood cells, express antigen on their cell surface. These antigens are recognised by antibodies and the cells are consequently destroyed by the immune response

E True — patients previously sensitised to mouldy hay react when spores are inhaled again. Typical sufferers of farmer's lung become breathless but not wheezy

BS17

A False — the fourth nerve is the trochlear nerve, the abducent nerve is the sixth

B False — the chorda tympani runs with the facial nerve but carries taste fibres of the ninth (glossopharyngeal) and eleventh (vagus) nerves

C False — a bulbar palsy causes fasciculation

D True — another cause is sarcoidosis

E False — the oculomotor nerve (third) supplies all the extraocular muscles except the lateral rectus (supplied by the sixth nerve) and the superior oblique (supplied by the fourth nerve)

BS18

A False — there is little alveolar development before 30–32 weeks

B True

C False — surfactant is produced by type 2 pneumocytes

D True — this is Potter sequence

E True

BS19

A True

B False — ADH secretion is reduced leading to increased urine production

C True — ADH release is also stimulated by pain and stress

D True — other drugs which stimulate ADH release include morphine, barbiturates and cholinergics

E False — this inhibits release and in turn leads to increased urine volume

BS20

A False — C3 is the most abundant

B True — phagocytic cells have receptors for C3b

C True — CRP is an acute phase protein

D False — it facilitates phagocytosis, the respiratory burst of neutrophils occurs later

E False — C3a and C5a complement fractions are anaphylatoxins and can directly stimulate mast cells to release further mediators of the inflammatory response such as histamine, tumour necrosis factor and kinins

BS21

A True — it is increased by anaemia, excitement or pyrexia

B True

C True — this is due to delayed closure of the stenosed aortic valve which thus occurs after pulmonary valve closure

D False — it is loud in mitral stenosis

E False — it occurs just before the first sound

BS22

A True — insulin also increases the rate of synthesis of glycogen and proteins

B False — insulin stimulates glycolysis

C False — insulin consists of two chains covalently joined by disulphide links

D True

E True — insulin signals that glucose is abundant and gluconeogenesis is therefore unnecessary

BS23

A True — this is a reflection of a generalised effect on protein synthesis and may explain, for instance, the increased glycolysis seen after thyroxine administration

B False — Na/K$^+$ ATPase is responsible for transport of these ions across membranes. It is fundamental in the maintenance of cellular homoestasis and as its name implies uses large amounts of ATP releasing heat in the process

C True — triglycerides and phospholipids are also reduced. In T4 deficiency the excess triglycerides may be implicated in the excessive arteriosclerosis that is characteristic of prolonged hypothyroidism

D True — mean blood pressure is largely unaffected because the pressor effects of T4 are balanced by reduced systemic vascular resistance and vasodilatation. These latter effects cause widening of the pulse pressure

E False — increased T4 feeds back to suppress TSH secretion

BS24

A True — also the uterus, small and large intestines, gall bladder and bronchioles

B False — this is lined by stratified squamous epithelium
C False — this is lined by stratified cuboidal epithelium
D True
E False — this is lined by simple squamous epithelium

BS25
A True — urine is excreted from 10 weeks onwards
B True — although the fetal kidney has a lobulated appearance this usually disappears before birth in term infants
C True — as do the renal calyces and collecting ducts
D True — the bladder forms from the ventral and cephalic portion of the cloaca after separation from the rectum
E False — nephrogenesis is complete at 36 weeks gestation, after this time the nephrons increase in size but not in number

BS26
A False — antibody-dependent complement activation is the classic pathway by which polyvalent C1q is linked with antibody and this activates in turn C4 and C2 forming C4b2b which has C3 convertase activity
B True — C3 is converted to a small molecule C3a and a larger molecule C3b
C True — the alternative pathway is triggered directly by the effect of microbial lipopolysaccharide on C3bBb. This causes the conversion of C3 to C3a and C3b and the consequent common pathway of complement activation is triggered
D True — C3a and C5a can independently activate neutrophils and cause mast cell degranulation
E False — C4b2b is the final component of the *classic* pathway before activation of C3, the first step of the common pathway

BS27
A False — meiosis is the nuclear division which gives rise to gametes
B False — human somatic cells contain 46 chromosomes consisting of 22 autosomal pairs plus sex chromosomes. In the basic haploid set $n = 23$ and after fertilisation the zygote contains a diploid set of chromosomes $2n = 46$
C False — in the polyploid state chromosome numbers are exact multiples of the haploid stage e.g. $3n$. In the aneuploid state

chromosome numbers are not exact multiples of the haploid stage e.g. $2n + 1$, as in trisomies

D False — a chimera is the presence of two different cell lines resulting from fusion of two zygotes e.g. 46XX/46XY, a true hermaphrodite. A mosaic is the presence of two different cell lines derived from one zygote

E True — uniparental disomy is the inheritance of both alleles of a gene from one parent only. Another example is Prader–Willi syndrome

BS28

A True

B False — about a third of the tidal volume is equivalent to the physiological dead space

C True

D False — this is the vital capacity

E False — this is the residual volume. Residual volume + vital capacity = total lung capacity

B29

A False — production starts in the later stages of pregnancy. Secretion usually starts on the first day

B False — the transition to mature breast milk takes 2–4 weeks

C False — 10–40 ml/day is usually produced

D True

E True — colostrum's chief benefit is immunological rather than nutritional

BS30

A True

B True — this causes post-synaptic neuronal discharges to decrease. The fatigue is due to depletion of the supply of stored transmitters such as acetylcholine

C False — acidosis suppresses neuronal excitability and can thus lead to coma. Increasing alkalosis however causes increased synaptic transmission and hence the occurrence of convulsions in alkalotic patients such as those with early salicylate poisoning or in patients who hyperventilate

D True — this so-called post-tetanic facilitation of response may double the post-synaptic response and may persist for hours in some neurons

E False — strychnine augments synaptic transmission by inhibiting inhibitory neurotransmitters

2: Cardiology

Answers to this section are to be found
between pages 22 and 26

QUESTIONS

C1 Causes of secondary hypertension include
A Addison's disease
B Neuroblastoma
C Turner's syndrome
D Porphyria
E Polyarteritis nodosa

C2 In coarctation of the aorta
A Fifty per cent of patients have additional cardiac anomalies
B The aortic valve is usually normal
C In young patients inequality of arm pulses may be evident even after repair
D Collateral circulation is well developed at birth
E Rib notching is best seen in the first and second ribs

C3 Pulmonary vascularity is increased in
A Tricuspid atresia
B Ebstein's disease
C Truncus arteriosus
D Hypoplastic left heart
E Coarctation of the aorta

C4 In transposition of the great vessels with an intact interventricular septum
A The blood in the aorta has a higher oxygen content than that in the left ventricle
B The infant fails a hyperoxia test
C The ECG is characteristically normal
D Continued patency of the ductus arteriosus should be ensured
E Tachyarrhythmias are very common following the arterial switch operation

C5 In a large patent ductus arteriosus (PDA)

A Presentation is usually in the first four months of life
B A systolic thrill is always present
C Infants may present with poor weight gain
D The second sound in the pulmonary area is split
E There is pulmonary hypertension

C6 The aortic arch

A Is interrupted in 10% of all cases of congenital heart disease
B May be abnormal in Di George syndrome
C Is in the posterior mediastinum
D Is developed from the fourth left pharyngeal arch
E In the fetus is linked to the pulmonary artery via the ductus arteriosus

C7 In aortic stenosis in childhood

A The lesion is usually secondary to rheumatic fever
B Subvalvular stenosis is associated with William's syndrome
C Calcification of the valve cusp starts in the first year of life
D A loud ejection click implies critical stenosis
E The heart is enlarged

C8 Heart failure occurs within the first few weeks of life in

A Truncus arteriosis
B Ebstein's disease
C Severe pulmonary stenosis with ASD
D Hypoplastic left heart
E Tricuspid atresia

C9 A venous hum

A Is abolished by lightly compressing the jugular venous system
B Is heard in the neck
C Is characteristically accentuated in late systole
D Is a common insignificant bruit
E Consists of a soft humming sound

C10 Congenital complete heart block

A Is associated with a higher ventricular rate than atrial rate
B Is associated with maternal thyroid disease

C Produces cannon 'a' waves in the JVP
D Has a good prognosis
E Is associated with transposition of the great vessels

C11 Atrial septal defects

A Have an RSR pattern in R chest leads
B Account for 10% of congenital heart defects
C Are frequently associated with supraventricular arrhythmias in childhood
D Are rarely associated with bacterial endocarditis
E Are usually of the ostium primum type

C12 In the normal heart

A The first sound is produced by closure of the aortic and pulmonary valves
B The second sound is due to closure of the atrioventricular valves
C The third sound is due to rapid filling of the ventricles during diastole
D The fourth sound is the result of atrial contraction causing a brief increase in flow into the left ventricle
E The fourth sound occurs just before the second sound

C13 Infective endocarditis

A Is most commonly due to *Streptococcus viridans*
B Following surgery is usually due to haemophilus
C Is more common in large cardiac defects
D Frequently occurs in ostium secundum atrial septal defects
E Is associated with splenomegaly

C14 Hypertension

A Causes 'cotton wool' exudates in the retina
B In adolescents is virtually always secondary hypertension
C That is associated with muscle cramps and polyuria suggests hyperaldosteronism
D Is a complication of Takayasu's arteritis
E Requires the use of as broad a cuff as possible for accurate measurement

C15 In tetralogy of Fallot

A Cyanosis may be absent at birth

B Hypercyanotic attacks may be treated with beta-blockers

C The degree of cyanosis is determined by the degree of overriding of the aorta

D The heart has a characteristic snowman appearance on chest X-ray

E The VSD is usually of the perimembranous type

ANSWERS

C1

A False — glucocorticoid deficiency causes hypotension. Cushing's disease is a cause of secondary hypertension

B True

C True — although coarctation of the aorta is the commonest cardiovascular lesion in Turner's syndrome it is not a constant finding

D True

E True — this illness often presents with renovascular lesions that show a necrotising vasculitis

C2

A True — VSDs, mitral valve anomalies and aortic stenosis are the commonest accompanying lesions

B False — the aortic valve is bicuspid in 70% of cases

C True — some coarctations are repaired with flaps of the left subclavian artery

D False — the coarcted area is not critical in the fetal circulation and there is no 'incentive' for development of collaterals. Neonatal presentation may occur when the ductus arteriosus closes and the systemic circulation is critically compromised

E False — notching of the inferior border of the ribs from pressure erosion by collateral vessels is often seen in late childhood but does not usually affect the upper or lower two to three ribs

C3

A False — in tricuspid atresia there is reduced pulmonary vascularity, a square-shaped heart and the pulmonary bay on chest X-ray is empty due to low flow in the pulmonary artery

B False — there is reduced pulmonary blood flow

C True

D True — there is increased pulmonary vascularity and pulmonary venous congestion due to poor left ventricular function

E True — there is increased pulmonary vascularity and pulmonary venous congestion due to systemic obstruction

C4

A False — blood in the left ventricle and the pulmonary artery has a higher oxygen content than that in the aorta

B True — the arterial oxygen does not rise appreciably when the child breathes 100% oxygen for 20 min

C True — the ECG shows normal neonatal right-sided dominance

D True — a prostaglandin E1 infusion temporarily maintains the patency of the ductus arteriosus until a balloon atrial septostomy (Rashkind procedure) is performed to allow mixing of oxygenated and deoxygenated blood in the atria

E False — following arterial switch sinus rhythm is usually maintained

C5

A True — in a large PDA infants usually present with poor weight gain and feeding problems in the first months of life

B False — a thrill is not always present

C True — feeding problems and poor weight gain are common

D False — the second sound is loud and single

E True — these individuals have severe pulmonary hypertension with the pulmonary pressure at or approaching systemic pressure

C6

A False — an interrupted aortic arch accounts for less than 1% of all cases of congenital heart disease

B True — there is often a right-sided or double aortic arch

C False — it is only in the superior mediastinum, the descending aorta is in the posterior mediastinum

D True

E True

C7

A False — the majority of cases in childhood are congenital

B False — in William's syndrome there is usually supravalvular aortic stenosis

C False — calcification may start in adolescence but rarely becomes important before the fifth decade in males and later in females

D False — when the aortic valve is mobile the murmur is preceded by an ejection click, the more severe the stenosis the closer the ejection click becomes to the first sound and the quieter it becomes

E False — the heart size is usually normal

C8

A True — the increased pulmonary blood causes dyspnoea and fatigue

B False — heart failure is rare in the first month

C False — heart failure is rare in the first month

D True — heart failure may occur in the first few days of life and is severe; most infants do not survive. Transplantation is an option but is limited due to infrequent availability of donor hearts

E False — heart failure does not occur in the newborn period

C9

A True

B True

C False — it is heard in both systole and diastole

D True

E True

C10

A False — the atria and ventricles beat independently of each other, but the atrial rate is higher

B False — it is associated with maternal connective tissue disorders, particularly systemic lupus erythematosus

C True — this is due to the right atrium contracting at times against a closed tricuspid valve

D True — most are asymptomatic and lead normal lives but if the heart rate is very slow dizziness or syncope occur and there is a risk of sudden death

E True — it may occur following surgery for tetralogy of Fallot, atrioventricular defects and ventricular septal defects

C11

A True — this is probably due to prolonged depolarisation of the hypertrophied right ventricular outflow tract. This hypertrophy is in response to chronic volume overload. The pattern is not specific for ASD and is found in 5–10% of normal children

B True

C False — atrial arrhythmias are rare in childhood

D True — endocarditis is very rare but some authorities still suggest antibiotic prophylaxis until the defect is closed and also after surgery if prosthetic material is used

E False — most are of the ostium secundum type

C12

A False — the first heart sound is due to closure of the atrioventricular tricuspid and mitral valves

B False — the second sound is caused by closure of the aortic and pulmonary valves

C True

D True — the third sound is generally thought to represent rapid ventricular filling. The fourth heart sound is caused by active atrial contraction

E False — the fourth sound is heard in late diastole just before the first heart sound

C13

A True — *Streptococcus viridans* is the commonest organism followed by *Staphylococcus aureus*

B False — the non-haemolytic staphylocci are more common after surgery

C False — small defects are more likely to develop endocarditis than larger ones

D False — endocarditis 'never' occurs in secundum defects and when it occurs in primum defects it is not the atrial septal defect which is affected but the abnormally cleft mitral valve

E True

C14

A True — longstanding hypertension causes hard exudates, haemorrhages and papilloedema

B False — in the older child or adolescent hypertension may be of the primary or essential type

C True

D True — bilateral renal artery stenosis may be a feature

E True — blood pressure should be measured with the child lying or sitting and with the sphygmomanometer at the level of the heart. The cuff should cover at least two-thirds of the upper arm. A narrow cuff gives falsely high results

C15

A True — postnatal changes may include increasing right ventricular outflow obstruction. Before this the shunt across the ventricular septal defect may be from left to right and the baby is therefore acyanotic

B True — however oxygen and correction of acidosis may be more urgently required

C False — the degree of pulmonary outflow obstruction determines the degree of right to left shunting across the ventricular septal defect

D False — the typical appearance is a boot-shaped heart with the apex lifted by right ventricular hypertrophy, an empty pulmonary bay due to the low volume of blood in the pulmonary artery, and a narrow pedicle due to the overriding aorta

E True

3: Dermatology

*Answers to this section are to be found
between pages 30 and 32*

QUESTIONS

D1 Naevus flammeus (port wine) lesions
A Develop at 2–3 weeks of age
B Occur in Rubinstein–Taybi syndrome
C Usually disappear by the age of 2 years
D Often have a unilateral distribution
E Are deep cystic lesions

D2 Erythema nodosum is associated with the following
A Streptococcal tonsillitis
B Leprosy
C Sulphonamides
D Psittacosis
E Vancomycin

D3 The mucous membrane is affected in
A Psoriasis
B Stevens–Johnson syndrome
C Lichen planus
D Herpes simplex virus infection
E Chickenpox

D4 With regard to vascular naevi
A Capillary haemangioma and limb hypertrophy occur in Klippel–
   Trenaunay–Weber syndrome
B Cavernous haemangioma are also known as 'stork marks'
C Cavernous haemangioma are usually present at birth
D Those which obscure the visual axis require treatment
E Thrombocytopenia occurs with large strawberry marks in
   Kasabach–Merritt syndrome

D5 Fabry's disease (angiokeratoma corporis diffusum)
A Is an X-linked recessive disorder
B Is associated with skin lesions which are most profuse on the face and scalp
C Is caused by beta-galactosidase deficiency
D May be dominated by renal and cardiac dysfunction in adults
E Is associated with mental retardation

D6 Light sensitivity in the neonatal period occurs in
A Xeroderma pigmentosa
B Hartnup disease
C Neonatal lupus erythematosus
D Incontinentia pigmenti
E Mastocytosis

D7 Pruritus occurs in
A Pinworm infestation
B Dermatitis herpetiformis
C Ehlers–Danlos syndrome
D Acute renal failure
E Hepatitis B infection

D8 In anhidrotic ectodermal dysplasia
A Inheritance is usually autosomal recessive
B The palmar skin is an appropriate site for a skin biopsy
C There are prominent low-set ears
D There is crowding of the teeth in the lower jaw
E Pilocarpine iontophoresis demonstrates increased sweating

D9 Diagnostic clues may be obtained from the nails in
A Fetal alcohol syndrome
B Hidrotic ectodermal dysplasia
C Iron deficiency
D Erythema nodosum
E Goldenhar syndrome

D10 Considering pigment disorders
A In Peutz–Jeghers syndrome melanotic macules are most prominent on the nose and nasal bridge

B In McCune–Albright syndrome *café-au-lait* spots usually have smooth borders
C Incontinentia pigmenti is lethal in females
D Chediak–Higashi syndrome presents with hyperpigmented patches on the buttocks
E Waardenburg syndrome is characterised by a white forelock

ANSWERS

D1

A False — these are present at birth

B True — they also occur in Beckwith–Wiedemann syndrome and Klippel–Trenaunay–Weber syndrome

C False — they change with maturation either becoming slightly raised or they may fade, but they do not disappear. They are a permanent skin defect

D True

E False — they consist of dilated dermal capillaries

D2

A True

B True

C True — another drug which is implicated is the contraceptive pill

D True — the granulomatoses of the lung such as tuberculosis, sarcoidosis and histoplasmosis are also associated with erythema nodosum

E False

D3

A False

B True — mucosal involvement may be severe

C True — mucosal involvement is frequent

D True

E True

D4

A True

B False — capillary haemangioma are known as 'salmon patches' or 'stork marks'

C False — these appear during the neonatal period but are rarely present at birth

D True — treatment may involve corticosteroids or interferon therapy

E True

D5

A True — it is fully penetrant in males and of variable penetrance in carrier females

B False — skin lesions are profuse over the genitalia, hips, buttocks and thighs, and in the umbilical and inguinal regions

C False — there is lysosomal alpha-galactosidase deficiency

D True — renal and cardiac involvement are the usual cause of death

E False

D6

A False — light sensitivity is rare in the neonatal period but may present with photophobia or erythema. If xeroderma pigmentosa is suspected avoidance of ultraviolet light is important in early childhood

B True — the use of phototherapy in neonates may make this disorder apparent at an early stage

C True

D False

E False

D7

A True — this causes pruritus ani

B True

C False — this is a connective tissue disorder

D False — pruritus occurs in chronic renal failure

E True — due to conjugated hyperbilirubinaemia

D8

A False — inheritance is X-linked recessive

B True

C True — the typical features include dry pale skin, sparse eyelashes, peg-like teeth and frontal bossing. Conductive deafness and atopy are also associated

D False — the teeth are widely spaced and 'peg-like'

E False — sweating is absent despite iontophoresis

D9

A True — small or hypoplastic nails occur

B True — nail changes are characteristic

C True — koilonychia or spoon-shaped nails are a feature
D False
E False — this is associated with preauricular skin tags, asymmetric
   facial hypoplasia, and cervical vertebral defects

D10
A False — the spots are prominent on the lips
B False — the edges are irregular and the patches are usually
   unilateral
C False — the disease is X-linked recessive and lethal in males
D False — this disorder of granule-containing cells affects white blood
   cells, melanosomes and Schwann cells. The melanosome defect
   causes partial albinism
E True — other features include heterochromia and deafness. It is
   inherited in an autosomal dominant fashion

4: ENT and Ophthalmology

Answers to this section are to be found between pages 36 and 39

QUESTIONS

EE1 In retinitis pigmentosa
A Night vision is preserved
B Arterial crowding is apparent
C There is an association with Peutz–Jeghers syndrome
D There may be confusion with Niemann–Pick disease
E Electroretinography (ERG) shows delayed retinal conduction

EE2 Otitis media
A In the neonate is caused by Gram-negative organisms in 20% of cases
B That causes perforation of the ear-drums may benefit from topical antibiotics
C Frequently occurs in children who swim while they have grommets *in situ*
D Is most commonly due to *Streptococcus pneumoniae*
E In children with Down's syndrome is more likely to be due to pseudomonas infection

EE3 With regard to the eye
A The lens of the newborn is more spherical than that of the adult
B Retinal haemorrhages in a newborn baby suggest peripartum asphyxia
C In the retina the cone receptor cells greatly outnumber the rod cells
D The canal of Schlemm drains fluid from the posterior chamber
E Six extraocular muscles in the orbit control eye movement

EE4 Deafness is a feature of the following syndromes
A Alport's syndrome
B Neurofibromatosis type 1
C Goldenhar syndrome

D Pendred's syndrome
E Tay–Sachs disease

EE5 Regarding nutritional disorders
A Riboflavin deficiency produces conjunctivitis
B Vitamin C deficiency may lead to gross proptosis
C Vitamin D levels are decreased by phenytoin therapy
D Night blindness is a late symptom of vitamin A deficiency
E Ptosis and nystagmus occur in vitamin B1 (thiamine) deficiency

EE6 Penetrating injuries to the eye should be suggested by the presence of
A Multiple retinal haemorrhages
B Pupillary irregularity
C Hypopyon
D Bilateral cataracts
E Fourth nerve palsy

EE7 Considering refractive errors
A Emmetropia is the condition where no refractive error is present
B Myopia is the commonest refractive error in infancy
C Hypermetropia is due to the eye being relatively long in its axial length
D Anisometropia is the condition where there is a significant difference in refraction between the two eyes
E Astigmatism may be corrected using a cylindric spectacle lens

EE8 Considering eye development
A Aniridia is associated with a chromosomal abnormality
B The orbital volume doubles in the first year of life
C Newborn babies may not produce tears when crying
D Failure of canalisation of the nasolacrimal duct results in conjunctivitis
E Colobomata may be inherited in an autosomal dominant fashion

EE9 With regard to the nose
A Epistaxis is associated with menarche
B Toxic shock syndrome is a complication of surgical packing of the nose

C The nasal secretions contain IgA

D Perforation of the nasal septum occurs in syphilis

E Nasal septal deviation is usually congenital

EE10 Regarding retinopathy of prematurity

A Normal angiogenesis is complete by 34 weeks

B The nasal retinal field is most often affected

C Cryotherapy may reduce complications

D In 90% of cases there is spontaneous arrest of disease process

E Painful blindness occurs

ANSWERS

EE1

A False — night blindness is a common presentation

B False — arterial attenuation and increased spacing are a feature. The typical appearance of the retina is described as salt and pepper retinitis

C False — retinitis pigmentosa is associated with Usher syndrome and retinitis pigmentosa like retinal degeneration occurs in several disorders including Laurence–Moon–Biedl syndrome, abetali-poproteinaemia and the mucopolysaccharidoses

D False — Niemann–Pick disease is a neurodegenerative storage disorder. Ophthalmic findings are a cherry red spot on the macula in 50% of cases

E True

EE2

A True

B True — the discharge may be cultured and appropriate systemic and local treatment planned

C False — the incidence of infection is very low. The use of earplugs is controversial

D True

E False

EE3

A True

B False — superficial retinal haemorrhages are often found in new-born infants and resolve spontaneously

C False — rod receptors outnumber cone receptors except at the macula

D False — they drain aqueous fluid from the anterior chamber

E True

EE4

A True — the commonest presentation is with asymptomatic micro-scopic haematuria. Sensorineural deafness is associated with this condition

B False — bilateral acoustic neuromas occur in neurofibromatosis
type 2
C False — abnormalities of the pinna and preauricular skin tags are
associated with facial hypoplasia and abnormalities of the cervical
spines
D True — this familial syndrome is congenital hypothyroidism and
deafness
E False — hyperacusis and a startle response are early features of
this condition

EE5

A True — cheilosis and seborrhoeic dermatitis are common results of
vitamin B2 deficiency
B True — spontaneous orbital haemorrhages can occur
C True — phenytoin disrupts vitamin D metabolism
D False — it is an early sign
E True — peripheral neuritis and myalgia are also associated with
dry beriberi

EE6

A False — such haemorrhages suggest shaking or asphyxia, as may
be found in child abuse
B True
C True — this is pus in the anterior chamber
D False — penetrating injuries are usually unilateral
E False
One must have a high suspicion for penetrating injuries, the
only symptom may be grittiness in the eye. X-ray films may
reveal radio-opaque objects but wood splinters or thorns are
radiolucent

EE7

A True
B False — hypermetropia (long-sightedness) is more common. Myopia (short-sightedness) may be familial and is more common in
preterm infants especially if they have retinopathy of prematurity
C False — in long-sightedness the anteroposterior diameter is relatively short

D True – this may cause amblyopia if left uncorrected. The Greek prefix 'aniso' means unequal and can also be applied to the pupil size – anisocoria

E True – astigmatism is due to irregularity of the cornea or lens. Children may try to overcome this with accommodation by frowning or squinting

EE8

A True – there may be a deletion on the short arm of chromosome 11

B True

C True – tears are often absent with crying until the age of 1–3 months

D False – a bacterially infected sticky eye is associated with conjunctivitis and erythema but these are absent if the collection of fluid is merely due to a blocked duct

E True – the finding of a coloboma should prompt full ocular examination looking for other defects

EE9

A True – there is no obvious explanation. The commonest cause of epistaxis is trauma, usually due to nose-picking

B True – toxic shock syndrome is most commonly due to *Staphylococcus aureus* toxins that may be in the nose or on the swab used

C True – IgA is the predominant immunoglobulin of the mucous membranes and the gastrointestinal tract

D True – a serosanguinous nasal discharge is found in 10% of early presentations of congenital syphilis. A saddle nose and nasal septal perforation are late signs

E False – congenital deviation and perforation are rare. Trauma and infections such as syphilis or tuberculosis are more usual causes

EE10

A False – angiogenesis proceeds from the disc to the periphery reaching the outer rim of the retina nasally at 36/40 and temporally by 40/40

B False – the area of the retina that is vascularised last is the most frequently involved and therefore the temporal fields are affected more often than the nasal fields

C True — cryotherapy may reduce the more severe complications of retinopathy of prematurity to some degree

D True — in less than 10% is there progression to severe disease

E True

5: Gastroenterology and Nutrition

Answers to this section are to be found
between pages 45 and 49

QUESTIONS

G1 Causes of hepatic cirrhosis in childhood include

A Wilson's disease

B Tyrosinaemia

C Hirschsprung's disease

D Gaucher's disease

E Phenylketonuria

G2 In malrotation of the intestine

A The diagnosis can be confidently confirmed on a plain abdominal film

B There is abnormal rotation around the inferior mesenteric artery

C The ligament of Treitz is positioned to the right on barium meal

D The mesenteric stalk is uncharacteristically wide

E Surgical correction fixes the caecum in the right iliac fossa

G3 Recognised features of coeliac disease include

A Hypersplenism

B Mouth ulcers

C Perifollicular haemorrhages

D Cataracts

E Intolerance to rice

G4 Meckel's diverticulum

A Is a vestige of the urachus

B Is present in 2% of the population

C May have ectopic gastric tissue

D Is characterised by painless rectal bleeding

E May be implicated in a Richter's hernia

G5 The following occur in kwashiorkor

A Poor appetite

B Moon face
C Preservation of hair
D Low circulating levels of cortisol
E Hypoplasia of the bone marrow

G6 Bilary atresia
A Is suggested by a family history of cholestatic jaundice
B Is characterized by bile-stained vomiting
C Has a characteristic pattern of uptake of the radioisotope imidodi-acetic acid (HIDA)
D Demands intraoperative cholangiography
E Most commonly affects ducts above the porta hepatis

G7 The following statements are true with regard to vitamins
A Vitamin D toxicity causes an elevated S–T segment
B Vitamin A deficiency is characterised by dry skin, hepatospleno-megaly, headache and joint pains
C Vitamin K is water soluble
D Vitamin E is found in high concentrations in animal tissues
E Vitamin C is ascorbic acid

G8 Constipation is caused by
A Cystic fibrosis
B Hyperthyroidism
C Hypocalcaemia
D Hyperkalaemia
E Renal tubular acidosis

G9 Ulcerative colitis in childhood
A Demonstrates extraintestinal manifestations more commonly than is the case in adults
B Is characterised by iritis early in the course of the disease
C Is associated with pyoderma gangrenosum
D Is associated with Turner's syndrome
E Accounts for 20% of all cases of ulcerative colitis

G10 Gastrointestinal manifestations of cystic fibrosis include
A Intestinal haemangiomas
B Biliary cirrhosis

C Intussusception
D Appendicitis
E Oesophageal reflux

G11 Causes of acute pancreatitis in childhood include
A Haemochromatosis
B Chickenpox
C Reye's syndrome
D Hypoparathyroidism
E Azathioprine

G12 The tongue
A Becomes red and then white in scarlet fever
B Is smooth in familial dysautonomia
C Is enlarged as part of generalised visceral enlargement in Beckwith–Wiedmann syndrome
D Is enlarged in hyperthyroidism
E If described as 'geographical' signifies underlying pathology

G13 In the oral mucosa
A Abnormal pigmentation occurs in Cushing's disease
B Palatal petechiae are characteristic in chickenpox
C Pigmented lines are seen near the dental margins of the gums in lead and mercury poisoning
D Freckling of the lips occurs in measles
E Herpes simplex virus infection is usually type 2

G14 Congenital chloridorrhoea
A Is inherited as an autosomal dominant condition
B Results from a defect in chloride/potassium transport in the ileum and colon
C Is associated with maternal oligohydramnios
D If not treated with appropriate electrolyte therapy may result in developmental delay
E Is associated with a metabolic alkalosis

G15 In viral hepatitis type B
A The presence of hepatitis B surface antibody (HBs Ab) indicates a highly infectious state

B The presence of hepatitis B core antibody (HBc Ab) IgM in high titre indicates past exposure to hepatitis B

C There may be associated papular acrodermatitis

D Only a small proportion of infections in early life are symptomatic

E Arthritis is associated with circulating immune complexes

G16 Duodenal obstruction

A Due to stenosis most commonly occurs distal to the ampulla of Vater

B Due to an annular pancreas is associated with a normal underlying duodenum

C Is associated with polyhydramnios

D Is associated in 70% of cases with Down's syndrome

E Has a typical X-ray appearance

G17 Cow's milk

A Has three times the protein concentration of human milk

B Has less casein than human milk

C Is an inadequate source of iron

D Empties more slowly from the stomach than human milk

E Is a common source of brucella infection

G18 The following may complicate anorexia nervosa

A Cardiac arrhythmias

B Congestive heart failure

C Hypertension

D Hypothermia

E Acne vulgaris

G19 Regarding nutritional deficiency states

A Pellagra is caused by riboflavin deficiency

B Vitamin C deficiency causes gingival haemorrhage

C Thiamine deficiency may cause cardiac failure

D Early vitamin A deficiency causes corneal clouding

E Folate deficiency is associated with coeliac disease

G20 Thiamine

A Is fat soluble

B Is present in nuts

C Is vitamin B2
D Deficiency causes pellagra
E Deficiency causes hoarseness due to paralysis of the laryngeal nerve

ANSWERS

G1

A True

B True — it is a feature of the chronic form of tyrosinaemia

C False

D False — usually the liver is involved only minimally

E False

G2

A False — a contrast film is required

B False — the axis of rotation is the superior mesenteric artery

C True

D False — the stalk may be very narrow and described as an 'apple-core mesentery'

E False — the large bowel is fixed in the left side of the peritoneal cavity and the small bowel in the right side

G3

A False — hyposplenism is a feature

B True — aphthous ulcers may be found in the mouth

C False — this is a feature of vitamin C deficiency

D False — cataracts are not a feature

E False — rice is well tolerated and is a major carbohydrate source

G4

A False — it is a vestige of the vitellointestinal duct

B True — the 'rule of twos' applies: a Meckel's diverticulum is present in 2% of the population, is 2 inches long and is located 2 feet from the ileocaecal junction

C True — this ectopic tissue may be subject to peptic ulceration and bleeding

D True

E False — an indirect inguinal hernia that contains a Meckel's diverticulum is termed a Littré's hernia. A Richter's hernia contains part of the bowel wall but does not cause obstruction

G5

A True

B True

C False — the hair is often sparse and thin. Dermatitis is common

D False — cortisol levels may be high, possible reflecting the catabolic state

E True

G6

A False — a family history of jaundice is a feature of 20% of cases of idiopathic neonatal hepatitis

B False — almost by definition the vomitus will not be bile-stained

C False — the isotope is taken up normally but its excretion into the duodenum is markedly impaired

D True

E True

G7

A True

B False — these are characteristic of vitamin A excess; deficiency causes photophobia, conjunctivitis, keratomalacia leading to blindness, defective tooth enamel, keratinization of mucous membranes and skin, and retarded growth

C False — vitamin K is fat soluble

D False — it is found in germ oils of various seeds, green leafy vegetables, nuts and legumes

E True

G8

A True — meconium ileus equivalent

B False — constipation occurs in hypothyroidism

C False — constipation occurs in hypercalcaemia

D False — constipation is seen in hypokalaemia

E True — possibly reflecting low potassium levels and poor smooth muscle activity in the intestine

G9

A False — extraintestinal manifestations are more common in adults but signs of arthritis are seen in about 10% of cases in childhood

B False — iritis develops relatively late in the course of the disease

C True

D True — the incidence is higher in whites, Jews, in the Northern hemisphere, in those with ankylosing spondylitis and those with Turner's syndrome

E True

G10

A False

B True — other hepatobiliary manifestations are lobular cirrhosis, cholelithiasis and biliary obstruction

C True — other intestinal manifestations include meconium ileus, rectal prolapse and distal intestinal obstruction syndrome

D False True ·

E True — recurrent coughing may increase intra-abdominal pressure and predispose to regurgitation of feeds

G11

A True — other causes include cystic fibrosis, diabetes mellitus, malnutrition, peptic ulcer, Kawasaki's syndrome

B False — viral infections implicated include Coxsackie B virus, Epstein–Barr virus, hepatitis A, influenza A, measles, mumps and rubella

C True

D False — it occurs in hyperparathyroidism

E True — other drugs implicated include methyldopa, tetracylines, thiazides and sulphonamides

G12

A False — it becomes white and coated and then red (a strawberry tongue)

B True — this is due to absence of papillae

C True

D False — macroglossia occurs in hypothyroidism

E False — this is benign and symptomless

G13

A False — abnormal pigmentation occurs in Addison's disease

B False — oral vesicles are found in chickenpox and palatal petechiae in rubella

C True — also in bismuth poisoning

D False — freckles occur in Peutz–Jeghers syndrome, Koplik's spots in measles

E False — it is usually type 1 and this is one of the most common infections involving the oral mucosa

G14

A False — it is inherited in an autosomal recessive fashion

B False — there is a defect in chloride/bicarbonate transport in the ileum and colon resulting in the loss of chloride in the stool. Sodium is also lost and secondary hyperaldosteronism may result

C False — there may be polyhydramnios with abdominal distension in the fetus. This may be detected on ultrasound

D True

E True — alkalosis is not present at birth but develops over subsequent weeks

G15

A False — this indicates immunity to hepatitis B, post-infective or with passive or active immunisation. The presence of HBe Ag suggests a highly infectious state

B False — a high titre suggests acute hepatitis, a low titre suggests chronic infection

C True

D True — 5% of infections in early infancy are symptomatic compared to 40% in later life

E True

G16

A True — in 90% of cases the obstruction is distal to the ampulla of Vater, this accounts for the bile-stained vomiting. Intrinsic obstruction may be by a web- or windsock-like diaphragm

B False — the duodenum is often stenosed or a diaphragm may be present

C True — because of failure to pass swallowed liquor to the lower gastrointestinal tract

D False — 30% of cases occur in Down's babies

E True — there is a classic 'double bubble' appearance caused by an enlarged air-filled stomach and air in the first part of the duodenum. After atresia, malrotation is the most common cause and should be sought by contrast studies

G17

A True
B False
C True
D True — bottle fed babies tend to sleep longer between feeds
E False

G18

A True — this may be due to hypokalaemia caused by vomiting
B True — dietary deficiencies may cause anaemia and vitamin deficiency states such as thiamine deficiency. This may cause heart failure
C False — hypotension and bradycardias are common
D True
E False — skin is usually dry and scaly. Lanugo hair is a feature

G19

A False — niacin deficiency causes pellagra. The classic skin changes are a photosensitive rash on the hands and feet and around the neck — 'Casal's necklace'
B True — this is a classic feature of scurvy. Other features include subperiosteal haemorrhages, fever, and poor wound healing
C True — so-called 'wet beriberi'
D False — the earliest sign is poor night vision. Corneal changes occur later
E True — folate is absorbed in the small bowel

G20

A False — it is water and alcohol soluble and fat insoluble
B True — it is also present in liver, pork, milk, whole grain cereals and wheat germ
C False — thiamine is vitamin B1. Riboflavin is vitamin B2
D False — deficiency causes beriberi, characterised by fatigue, irritability, anorexia, constipation, headache, insomnia, tachycardia, polyneuritis, and cardiac failure. Wernicke's encephalopathy also occurs
E True — this is a characteristic sign

6: Genetics

Answers to this section are to be found
between pages 53 and 55

QUESTIONS

GE1 The following conditions are autosomal dominant disorders
A Myotonic dystrophy
B Adult polycystic kidney disease
C Facioscapulohumeral dystrophy
D Diastrophic dwarfism
E Becker's muscular dystrophy

GE2 Regarding patterns of inheritance
A In an X-linked dominant disorder an affected father transmits the disease only to his daughters
B In an autosomal dominant disorder the chance of an affected parent having an affected child is 50% for each pregnancy
C In an X-linked recessive disorder each daughter of a carrier has a 25% chance of being a carrier herself
D In X-linked dominant disorders female patients have less severe manifestations
E In mitochondrial inheritance affected females cannot have affected sons

GE3 XYY males
A Have hypogonadism
B Are more likely than XY males to have problems with language development
C Often have severe nodulocytic acne
D Have an increased risk of developing hypothyroidism
E Are found in mental or penal institutions more often than expected from birth incidence

GE4 In Noonan's syndrome
A The karyotype is normal
B The cardiac defect is usually coarctation of the aorta

C Puberty frequently occurs early
D Cryptorchidism is frequent in males
E Tall stature commonly occurs

GE5 In Down's syndrome due to translocation
A Incidence is independent of maternal age
B Carrier mothers may have carrier children
C Paternal translocation carriers rarely have children with Down's syndrome
D A normal karyotype may be found in a phenotypic Down's baby
E IQ scores are higher than in cases of non-disjunction

GE6 The following statements are true with regard to genetic abnormalities
A Terminal deletion of 5p occurs in *cri du chat* syndrome
B A balanced translocation usually leads to an abnormal phenotype
C An unbalanced translocation may lead to spontaneous abortion
D Fragile X syndrome is associated with mental retardation
E Pericentric inversions of chromosomes usually lead to a normal phenotype

GE7 X-linked recessive disorders include
A Incontinentia pigmenti
B Duchenne muscular dystrophy
C Lesch–Nyhan syndrome
D Vitamin D resistant rickets
E Menkes' (kinky hair) syndrome

GE8 In Down's syndrome
A There is increased risk of atlantoaxial instability
B Twenty per cent of adults are hypothyroid
C Females may be fertile
D The recurrence risk to a mother with non-disjunction is 1%
E There is an increased incidence of leukaemia

GE9 The following statements are true with regard to inheritance
A Webbed toes has been postulated as a Y-linked condition
B Inborn errors of metabolism are usually inherited via the autosomal dominant route

C X-linked dominant conditions give rise to the disorder in hemi-
zygous males
D Tay–Sachs is usually due to a new gene mutation
E X-linked recessive disorders cannot be transmitted by a healthy
male

GE10 In fragile X syndrome
A The fragile site is on the short arm of the X chromosome
B Adult males are short in stature
C Macro-orchidism occurs in adult males
D The likelihood of finding fragile sites in carrier females recedes
with age
E Microcephaly is unusual

ANSWERS

GE1

A True

B True

C True

D False — this is inherited as an autosomal recessive condition

E False — this is inherited as an X-linked recessive condition

GE2

A True — an affected father transmits the affected X to his daughters and only unaffected Y chromosomes to his sons

B True — examples include Huntington's chorea and hereditary spherocytosis

C False — the risk is 50%

D True

E False — affected females may have affected sons and daughters. Affected males have normal children. Mitochondrially inherited disorders are only inherited from female patients

GE3

A False — this is in contrast to Klinefelter males (46,XXY)

B True — hearing and social skills are poorer

C True

D False

E True — the rate is twenty times that expected from the birth frequency of XYY of 1 in 1000 newborn males

GE4

A True — the phenotype in both males and females resembles Turner's syndrome

B False — pulmonary valve stenosis is the most characteristic cardiac finding

C False — puberty is usually delayed

D True

E False — short stature is characteristic

GE5

A True — this is in contrast to the non-disjunctional type where there is increased incidence with maternal age

B True

C True — there is a higher incidence if the mother carries the translocation

D True — the baby may be a mosaic with a low frequency of mosaic cells or have a 'hidden' translocation

E False — the IQ is not dependent on the type of chromosomal lesion

GE6

A True

B False — balanced translocations usually cause no phenotypical abnormality

C True — there is also an increased incidence of physical and mental handicaps in unbalanced translocations

D True — the phenotype is of developmentally delayed males with macro-orchidism, large ears and a 'lantern-like' prominent mandible

E True — no genetic material is inserted or deleted

GE7

A False — this is an X-linked dominant disorder

B True

C True

D False — this is an X-linked dominant disorder

E True

GE8

A True — anaesthetists may be wary of anaesthetising children with Down's syndrome

B True

C True

D True — this is also the risk to a 37-year-old mother of having an affected child

E True — the Philadelphia chromosome involves a 21-9 translocation. Early dementia of Alzheimer's type is a feature also

GE9

A True — this inheritance pattern has also been suggested for porcupine skin and hairy ears

B False — most single enzyme defects are inherited as autosomal recessive conditions

C True

D False — it is usually inherited in an autosomal recessive fashion

E True

GE10

A False — it is near the end of the long arm of the X chromosome

B True — as children those with fragile X are taller than other children but they do not achieve growth predicted by centile charts and adult males tend to be short

C True — 80% of adult fragile X males have macro-orchidism and 15% of prepubertal males

D True — fragile sites are only found in 50% of obligatory female carriers and the frequency of expression of fragile sites decreases with age

E True — many have a head circumference greater than the 97th centile

7: Growth and Endocrinology

*Answers to this section are to be found
between pages 60 and 64*

QUESTIONS

GR1 In Turner's syndrome

A Inheritance is autosomal dominant

B Congenital scleroderma is a common clue to the diagnosis

C Infertility is universal in untreated cases

D Gastrointestinal bleeding is a recognised association

E FSH levels are low in infancy

GR2 True precocious puberty (gonadotrophin-dependent) occurs in

A Hydrocephalus

B Untreated primary hypothyroidism

C Granulosa-theca cell ovarian tumours

D Congenital adrenal hyperplasia

E Hypothalamic hamartoma

GR3 In males

A The first sign of puberty is usually the appearance of pubic hair

B Puberty begins earlier than in girls

C Enlargement of the testis occurs before lengthening of the penis

D Peak height velocity occurs at pubic hair stage 3–4

E The haematocrit varies directly with Tanner stage

GR4 In incomplete (partial) precocious puberty

A Premature menarche is associated with elevated levels of gonado-
tropins

B Premature adrenarche is more common in the male than the
female

C The term premature thelarche is defined by breast development
before the age of 2 years in girls

D Hair appears first in the axilla in premature adrenarche

E Premature thelarche is often familial

GR5 In congenital adrenal hyperplasia

A Hyperkalaemia is a characteristic finding
B Early measurements of 17-hydroxyprogesterone acetate may be in the normal range
C Cortisol levels may be normal in the non-salt-losing type
D Steroid replacement may be discontinued at puberty
E Recognition is more easily achieved in males

GR6 In pseudohypoparathyroidism

A Arachnodactyly is a feature
B Parathyroid hormone (PTH) levels are normal
C Neonatal cataracts are a feature
D Phosphaturia occurs to a lesser degree than normal in response to PTH administration
E There is an association with thyroid hormone abnormalities

GR7 In testicular feminisation

A Ambiguous genitalia are found
B The testes are histologically normal
C The diagnosis may be made in 30% of girls with inguinal hernias
D Testosterone production is at approximately normal levels
E Rudimentary fallopian tubes may be found

GR8 In constitutional growth delay in boys

A Bone age is significantly delayed compared to chronological age
B Growth hormone levels are reduced
C T4 levels are reduced
D Testosterone administered intramuscularly accelerates height growth but not pubertal development
E There is a lower incidence than in girls

GR9 Gynaecomastia occurs in

A XYY karotype
B Methyldopa therapy
C Klinefelter's syndrome
D Testicular tumours
E Normal puberty

GR10 Gonadotropin-dependent precocious puberty
A Is commoner in females
B Results in giantism
C Results in advanced dental age
D Is associated with a brisk rise in LH levels following LHRH administration
E Should prompt cerebral imaging studies

GR11 Regarding normal growth in both males and females
A The jaw changes in configuration at puberty
B At birth the brain weighs approximately 50% of adult brain weight
C Human growth patterns differ considerably from those of other high primates
D Lymphoid tissue mass is greatest before adolescence
E Girls grow faster than boys from 1–4 years of age

GR12 In females
A The rate of growth during the pubertal growth spurt is faster than at any other time in extrauterine life
B Menarche occurs at Tanner stage 5 in 95%
C The development of a breast bud is the first sign of puberty
D Tanner staging of pubic hair is classified as stages 1–3
E Alkaline phosphatase levels vary with physical maturity

GR13 Cranial diabetes insipidous
A Results from an excess of antidiuretic hormone (ADH)
B That is caused by a head injury may not present immediately
C May appear in childhood in an autosomal dominant form
D Is associated with septo-optic dysplasia
E May be described as idiopathic in a large proportion of cases following investigations

GR14 Turner's syndrome is associated with
A Horseshoe kidneys
B Recurrent otitis media
C Ptosis
D Obstructive sleep apnoea
E Clinodactyly

GR15 Causes of short stature include

A Zinc deficiency

B Renal tubular acidosis

C Gilbert's syndrome

D Obstructive sleep apnoea

E Pseudohypoparathyroidism

ANSWERS

GR1

A False — this condition occurs sporadically. The typical genotype is 45XO but 30% of cases are mosaics

B False — this is not a diagnostic clinical manifestation. Congential lymphoedema is a common finding

C False — fertility has been reported in some individuals with Turner's syndrome

D True — abdominal pain, tenesmus or bloody diarrhoea suggest associated inflammatory bowel disease; recurrent gastrointestinal bleeding suggests gastrointestinal telangiectasia, also associated with Turner's syndrome

E False — FSH levels are high in infancy, with a progressive decrease in levels occuring at 2–3 years, eventually rising again to castrate adult levels by 10–11 years

GR2

A True — precocious puberty may be classified as true precocious puberty or precocious pseudopuberty. True precocious puberty is always isosexual and involves hypothalamic–pituitary–gonadal activation, with increased size and activity of the glands and development of secondary sexual characteristics. In precocious pseudopuberty some secondary sex characteristics appear but the gonads do not mature and there is no hypothalamic–pituitary–gonadal activation

B True

C False — this causes gonadotropin-independent precocious pseudo-puberty

D False — this also causes gonadotropin-independent precocious pseudopuberty

E True

GR3

A False — the first sign is usually testicular enlargement

B False — girls begin to develop on average 2 years before boys

C True — enlargement of the testis is followed by lengthening of the penis and then by the appearance of pubic hair

D True — peak height velocity in boys is at Tanner pubic hair stage 3–4 and in girls at pubic hair stage 2–3

E True — many types of laboratory data are uninterpretable without knowledge of the person's pubertal staging

GR4

A False — gonadotropin levels are normal

B False — it is much more frequent in females. The normal rise of androgens in mid-childhood manifests itself in this condition by the appearance of some pubic, and less commonly axillary hair, without breast development but with an increase in height velocity

C True

D False — hair appears first on the labia majora

E False — it is usually sporadic and rarely familial

GR5

A True — in salt-losers profound hyponatraemia and acidosis may also occur

B True — early postnatal levels are usually raised in normal babies. Levels that are raised at 24 h are usually abnormal

C True — the levels of cortisol in salt-losers are low

D False — treatment is lifelong. With intercurrent illness intravenous hydrocortisone may be necessary

E False — boys may appear relatively normal with moderate penile and testicular enlargement and scrotal rugosity. Affected females are more easily detected due to the clitoromegaly and scrotolabial folds

GR6

A False — short fingers are a characteristic finding, especially the fourth and fifth metacarpals ᴜˢ²⁰

B False — the levels are high and this distinguishes true hypothyroidism from pseudohypoparathyroidism. Administered PTH fails to increase serum calcium or decrease phosphate

C False — neonatal tetany is a common presentation and family history is positive in 50% of cases

D True — PTH normally causes an increase of phosphaturia in normal patients and hypoparathyroid patients

E True — TSH levels are raised and thyrotrophin-releasing hormone stimulation causes an exaggerated rise of TSH

GR7

A False — this is an extreme form of failure of virilisation of genetic males who appear female and have female genitalia at birth. They have a blind-ending vagina and absent uterus. Presentation is often delayed until after puberty when menarche fails to occur

B False — the testes are usually intra-abdominal and consist largely of seminiferous tubules

C False — 1–2% of girls with an inguinal hernia have this disorder

D True — the testes of affected adults produce normal male levels of testosterone

E True

GR8

A True — bone age is 1–4 years retarded

B False — all laboratory data should be normal

C False

D False — testosterone accelerates height and pubertal development

E False — constitutional delay occurs in both sexes, but fewer girls are referred for a medical opinion

GR9

A False — it occurs in Klinefelter's syndrome (47,XXY)

B True

C True

D True

E True — during pubertal development about 65% of boys develop varying degrees of temporary gynaecomastia. It may be asymmetrical

GR10

A True — no causative factor is found in 80–90% of girls. Gonadotropin-dependent precocious puberty is true precocious puberty

B False — final stature is short as an increased ossification rate results in early epiphyseal closure

C False — both dental and mental age are similar to chronological age, in contrast to the advanced bone age

D True — plasma LH and FSH levels are either elevated or within the normal range and following LHRH administration a response similar to that seen in normal puberty occurs

E True — a CT scan or MRI scan should be done to rule out a cerebral lesion such as a tumour

GR11

A True — the jaw becomes longer and the chin more pointed

B False — at birth the brain is 25% of its adult weight and at age 10 it is 95% of adult weight

C False — the characteristic shape of the human growth curve is shared by monkeys and apes

D True — lymphoid tissue reaches its maximum mass before adolescence and then declines to its adult size, probably under the direct influence of sex hormones

E True — at birth boys grow slightly faster than girls but from age 7 months to 4 years girls grow faster. From 4 years until puberty growth velocity is identical in both sexes

GR12

A True

B False — menarche usually occurs by late stage 3, but in 5% it does not occur until stage 5

C True — the appearance of a firm disc of tissue beneath the areola is followed by the appearance of pubic hair

D False — it is classified at stages 1–5 (see below)

E True — this rises to a peak at the period of peak height velocity, reflecting bone metabolic activity

With regard to pubic hair the Tanner stages are as follows:
stage 1 — preadolescent
stage 2 — sparse, lightly pigmented, straight hair on the medial border of labia
stage 3 — darker hair, beginning to curl, increased in amount
stage 4 — coarse, curly, abundant hair but less than adult amount
stage 5 — adult triangle, spread to medial surface of thighs

With regard to breast development the Tanner stages are as follows:
stage 1 — preadolescent

stage 2 — areolar diameter increased with breast and papilla elevated as small mound

stage 3 — breast and areola enlarged

stage 4 — areola and papilla form secondary mound

stage 5 — mature breast with nipple projecting and areola forming part of general breast contour

GR13

A False — it results from a lack of ADH

B True — after a head injury diabetes insipidus may occur immediately or after a delay of several months

C True — onset may be from birth to several years of age. The severity may vary within an individual over a period of time and it may vary within different family members

D True

E False — the cause of diabetes insipidus is often not found initially, but eventually only 20% are classified as idiopathic

GR14

A True — there may also be abnormal renal arteries and collecting systems

B True — it is also associated with Hashimoto's thyroiditis, glucose intolerance and multiple pigmented naevi

C True — other facial abnormalities include micrognathia, rotated ears, high arched palate and epicanthic folds

D False — this is not associated with Turner's syndrome

E True — short fourth and fifth metacarpals also occur along with classical cubitus valgus

GR15

A True — short stature may be caused by other nutritional deficiencies, abnormalities of digestion or problems with utilisation or retention of calories

B True

C False — this does not affect stature

D True

E True — other endocrine and metabolic causes include hypopituitarism, hypothyroidism and rickets

8: Haematology and Oncology

*Answers to this section are to be found
between pages 69 and 73*

QUESTIONS

H1 Wilms' tumours
A Of the rhabdoid type are considered to have favourable histology
B Are associated with a deletion on chromosome 11
C Of the familial form are usually unilateral
D Are associated with raised plasma renin levels
E Metastasise to the lungs

H2 Thrombocytopenia occurs in
A Kawasaki's disease
B Wiskott–Aldrich syndrome
C Aspirin therapy
D Scurvy
E Hypothermia

H3 The following statements regarding Ewing's sarcoma are correct
A The pelvis is commonly involved
B The central nervous system is the most common site of metastases
C Radiotherapy is ineffective
D The peak incidence is in the 1–5 year age group
E Disease involving the distal extremity shows the most favourable prognosis

H4 Glucose-6-phosphate dehydrogenase (G6PD) deficiency
A Results in an increase in reduced glutathione
B Is X-linked
C May require exchange transfusion in the neonatal period
D May cause crisis on consumption of paracetamol
E May cause crisis on consumption of chick peas

H5 Haemolytic anaemia

A Due to pyruvate kinase deficiency may present as jaundice in the neonatal period

B Occurs in hereditary spherocytosis

C Due to hereditary elliptocytosis is often asymptomatic

D Due to glucose-6-phosphate dehydrogenase deficiency causes haematuria

E May be treated operatively, preferably after the age of 10 years

H6 In Langerhans cell histocytosis (LCH)

A Boney lesions are punched out with evidence of reactive bone formation

B An eczematous rash occurs in 50% of cases

C Resolution may be spontaneous

D The histological features are the most important prognostic factors

E Older patients do best

H7 Aplastic anaemia

A Of the Faconi type is associated with X-linked inheritance

B In Schwachman–Diamond syndrome is accompanied by pancreatic insufficiency

C Due to Blackfan–Diamond syndrome presents in adolescence

D Occurs in paroxysmal nocturnal haemoglobinuria

E Is associated with streptomycin therapy

H8 Regarding brain tumours

A Astrocytomas typically seed throughout the neuroaxis

B Brain stem gliomas rarely present with raised intracranial pressure as an early sign

C In children less than 1 year there is an adult-like distribution of tumour sites

D The tissue of origin of a craniopharyngioma is neuroectodermal

E Unilateral cerebellar tumours cause ipsilateral signs

H9 Regarding anaemia in childhood

A Vitamin B12 deficiency is the commonest cause of childhood anaemia

B Proven iron deficiency merits full investigation of causes of haemorrhage as a first step

C Phenytoin therapy may be contributory
D In Crohn's disease anaemia is usually due to iron deficiency
E Anaemia due to Lesch–Nyhan syndrome is megaloblastic

H10 Neuroblastoma
A Arises in the thoracic cavity in 20% of cases
B Is commonly associated with hypertension
C Is suggested by high levels of urinary vanillyl mandelic acid (VMA)
D Which presents at less than 1 year has a better prognosis than those which present at an older age
E Stage 4S disease is defined as localised primary tumour with positive local nodes and spreads to liver, skin and bone marrow

H11 In hereditary spherocytosis
A An autosomal recessive mode of inheritance is most common
B The osmotic fragility of spherocytes is lower than that of normal RBCs
C Immature red cells show characteristic dysmorphic features
D The blood film may be confused with microangiopathic haemolytic anaemia
E Persistent splenomegaly occurs

H12 In von Willebrands disease
A Prothrombin time is normal
B Mucocutaneous bleeding is the predominant problem
C Inheritance is autosomal recessive
D Bleeding time is prolonged
E The incidence is as common as haemophilia A

H13 Common acute lymphoblastic leukaemia (ALL) is characterised by the following immunohistochemical results
A Surface immunoglobulin positivity
B PAS positivity
C CD10 negativity
D Sudan black negativity
E Cytoplasmic immunoglobulin positivity

H14 In the treatment of the leukaemias
A Vincristine encephalopathy is unrelated to dose

B Ptosis and sixth nerve palsies occur with vincristine
C Children should be excluded from school when neutropaenic
D Post-irridation somnolence syndrome occurs 1–2 months after completion of irridation
E Fungal infections such as aspergillosis or candidiasis produce easily distinguishable CT appearances

H15 Hereditary haemorrhagic telangiectasia (Osler–Weber–Rendu disease)
A Commonly causes epistaxis
B Is inherited as an autosomal dominant trait
C Decreases in severity with age
D Causes megaloblastic anaemia
E Is associated with disordered coagulation

ANSWERS

H1

A False — rhabdoid histology is unfavourable as are anaplasia and clear cell sarcoma, they account for 10% of cases and 60% of mortality

B True — in association with aniridia and Beckwith–Wiedmann syndrome

C False — familial tumours are usually bilateral

D True — this may be due to a pressure effect on the renal artery

E True — haematogenous spread to the lungs is common

H2

A False — thrombocytosis is a typical feature

B True — this condition is X-linked recessive and is characterised by severe eczema, thrombocytopenia and immunological deficiency

C False — this causes inhibition of prostaglandin synthetase and impaired thromboxane A_2 synthesis. It does not cause thrombocytopenia

D False — scurvy causes non-thrombocytopenic purpura and haemorrhages

E True — this is due to splenic sequestration

H3

A True — the most common sites are the pelvis, proximal humerus and proximal femur, but any bone can be involved

B False — the most common sites for metastases are the lungs

C False — Ewing's sarcoma are radiosensitive, primary treatment is with chemotherapy to control dissemination, but local control is achieved with radiotherapy

D False — the peak age is 10–15 years and there is a slight male predominance

E True — distal extremity disease has the most favourable prognosis whilst pelvic and sacral sites of tumour have a poor prognosis

H4

A False — G6PD maintains glutathione in its reduced state, so protecting red cell membranes from oxidant stress

B True

C True — neonatal jaundice is more common if infections or acidosis occur or if oxidant drugs are given to the neonate or the mother in late pregnancy

D False — drugs associated with haemolysis in G6PD deficiency include sulphonamides, nitrofurantoins, primaquine, chloramphenicol and naphthaquinolones

E False — the fava bean is the classic culprit

H5

A True — at other times infection may precipitate severe haemolysis

B True

C True — most cases are asymptomatic or have very mild chronic haemolysis requiring no further therapy

D True — haemoglobin and urobilinogen darken the urine. Tubular damage and renal dysfunction may occur

E True — splenectomy should be avoided in the first 10 years of life when the risk of post-splenectomy sepsis is highest. Splenectomy does not correct the underlying abnormality

H6

A False — classically the lesions are punched out lytic lesions with little sclerotic reaction

B False — the rash is usually like a seborrhoeic dermatitis

C True

D False — the degree of organ impairment is most important

E True — the best prognosis is in those over 2 years with no evidence of organ involvement

H7

A False — it shows autosomal recessive inheritance

B True

C False — this usually presents in infancy, 95% of cases occur before 2 years of age

D True — there is a disorder of red cells, white cells and platelets wherein they fix excessive amounts of complement with consequent cell lysis

E True — other drugs which are associated with aplastic anaemia include chloramphenicol, barbiturates, cimetidine and thiazides

H8

A False — they usually present with a mass effect such as obstructive hydrocephalus

B True — cranial nerve palsies and brain stem signs are more common

C True — over 2 years infratentorial tumours account for 60% of cases

D True — they are thought to arise from remnants of Rathke's pouch

E True — this is because of the double decussation of the cerebellar outflow tracts

H9

A False — iron deficiency anaemia is by far the most common

B False — iron deficiency is usually dietary in origin

C True — megaloblastic anaemia may occur

D False — Crohn's disease may affect the terminal ileum and hence intrinsic factor B12 complex absorption. A mixed picture is more common than iron or B12 deficiency anaemia

E True

H10

A True — these children may be picked up incidentally on chest X-ray or because of a Horner's syndrome

B False — hypertension is more commonly a feature of phaeochromocytoma tumours

C True

D True — older patients tend to have more disseminated disease

E False — 4S disease suggests a tumour localised to one side of the midline with one remote site such as skin, liver or marrow. Stage 1 disease is unilateral disease confined to the organ of origin; stage 2 is extension from organ of origin with or without local nodes but not beyond the midline; stage 3 extends beyond the midline with bilateral nodes and stage 4 is where there is remote disease

H11

A False — inheritance is autosomal dominant

B False — the cells are more vulnerable to osmotic changes than normal cells

C False
D True — the cells may appear fragmented on blood film but previous episodes and family history may aid the diagnosis
E True

H12
A True — the thrombin time and fibrinogen levels are normal and the partial thromboplastin time is prolonged
B True
C False — it is autosomal dominant
D True — the bleeding time is usually grossly prolonged
E False — haemophilia A is the commonest hereditary bleeding disorder

H13
A False — this is a feature of differentiated B-cell leukaemia or a B-cell leukaemia/lymphoma
B True
C False — CD10 is the typical positive marker in common ALL
D True — Sudan black is a marker of myeloid cells
E False — the presence of cytoplasmic immunoglobulin is more typical of a more differentiated pre-B ALL

H14
A True
B True — a peripheral symmetrical distal neuropathy is more common
C True — home tutoring may need to be considered
D True
E False — in immunocompromised patients the presentation and radiological findings are often atypical due to the poor host response to infection

H15
A True
B True
C False — telangiectasias become more evident with age and the patients become increasingly symptomatic

D False — chronic gastrointestinal blood loss usually causes iron deficiency anaemia

E False — the poor collagen support of the blood vessels means that haemostasis is poor but there is no defect of the coagulation cascade or platelet function

9: Immunology and Infections

*Answers to this section are to be found
between pages 79 and 84*

QUESTIONS

IN1 Lyme disease
A Is characterised by erythema ab igne
B Is caused by a spirochete, *Borrelia burgdorferi*
C Has a more severe and protracted course in patients with HLA DR-2
D Should be treated with tetracycline in young children
E Has late manifestations which occur weeks to months after the initial illness

IN2 Acute graft-versus-host disease
A Occurs up to 100 days post-transplant
B Causes a psoriasiform rash
C May cause obliterative bronchiolitis
D Is characterized by a swinging fever
E Is caused by reaction of donor lymphocytes versus host cell antigens

IN3 Wiskott–Aldrich syndrome
A Is inherited in an X-linked fashion
B Causes thrombocytosis
C Causes raised IgE levels
D Is associated with eczema
E Causes lymphopenia

IN4 In chronic granulomatous disease (CGD)
A The neutrophils fail to produce hydrogen peroxide (H_2O_2)
B The inheritance may be X-linked
C The polymorphs fail to reduce nitrazolium blue
D Neutrophil phagocytosis is normal
E Catalase-positive organisms cause most significant infections

IN5 Live vaccines include

A Cholera

B Pertussis

C Typhoid

D MMR

E BCG

IN6 In roseola infantum (exanthem subitum)

A Those affected are usually in their first years of school

B High fever occurs

C The rash appears as fever settles

D The child looks very unwell

E Desquamation generally occurs

IN7 Measles

A Is a DNA virus

B Is a common subclinical infection

C Transmission is via the oro-faecal route

D Is most infectious when the rash first appears

E Has a rash which starts on the chest and abdomen

IN8 Pseudomonas species

A Are Gram-negative bacilli

B Are sensitive to benzylpenicillin

C Frequently cause chronic sinusitis in cystic fibrosis patients

D If found in a sputum sample should suggest immunodeficiency

E Often cause otitis externa in normal children

IN9 The MMR vaccine

A May be used in the control of outbreaks of measles

B Is suitable for prophylaxis following exposure to mumps

C Is associated with parotid swelling in the 3rd week post-vaccination

D Should not be given to a child who has had single antigen measles
vaccine

E Is contraindicated in children receiving immunosuppressive therapy

IN10 Listeriosis

A Is caused by Gram-positive bacilli

B Acquired transplacentally frequently leads to abortion

C In the neonatal period usually presents as meningitis
D Is usually contracted from eating undercooked pork
E Is most effectively treated with erythromycin

IN11 The following are notifiable infectious diseases
A Smallpox
B Ophthalmia neonatorum
C Herpangina
D Roseola infantum
E Mumps

IN12 In congenital agammaglobulinaemia
A Lymphadenopathy and splenomegaly occur
B Maternal antibodies protect infants until about 6 months of age
C IgM levels are preserved
D Serial pulmonary function testing is indicated
E Presentation may be delayed until adolescence

IN13 In immunodeficiency diseases
A Thrombocytopenia occurs in Wiskott–Aldrich disease
B Di George syndrome is associated with congenital hepatitis
C Arthritis is a prominent clinical feature in X-linked agammaglo-
bulinaemia
D IgA deficiency may cause recurrent diarrhoea
E Severe combined immunodeficiency (SCID) may be treated with
bone marrow transplantation

IN14 Cholera
A Is due to a Gram-positive organism
B Has cattle as a reservoir of infection
C Involves the large intestine most severely
D Has an incubation period of 7–10 days
E Vaccine prevents the development of an asymptomatic carrier
state

IN15 With regard to staphylococcal infections
A *Staphylococcus albus* is responsible for the overwhelming majority of
skin infections
B A positive culture from a superficial site indicates infection

C Twenty per cent of adults are asymptomatic carriers
D Pneumonia usually follows a viral illness
E Symptoms of food poisoning usually occur after 10–12 h

IN16 Osteomyelitis

A That starts haematogenously begins as a metaphyseal abscess
B Is more likely to cause a septic arthritis in the neighbouring joint in older rather than younger children
C Due to salmonella species is more common in sickle cell patients
D Is reflected by positive blood cultures in 50–60% of cases of acute or subacute infections
E Of vertebrae should not be confused with discitis in adolescents

IN17 In children with congenital HIV infection

A Hepatosplenomegaly is common in the neonatal period
B DPT (diphtheria, pertussis, tetanus) vaccine should be withheld
C The oral polio vaccine is given as normal
D p24 antigen detection is generally considered proof of infection
E There is an increase in the ratio of helper (CD4$^+$) to suppressor (CD8$^+$) T cells

IN18 In cases of subacute sclerosing panencephalitis (SSPE)

A Rural children are more susceptible than urban children
B The measles infection was usually acquired before 18 months of age
C Measles virus may be recoverable from brain tissue biopsy
D Patients have usually had an encephalitic illness at the time of measles infection
E IgG and IgM versus the matrix (M) protein are found in the CSF

IN19 Nocardia infection

A Suggests underlying immunosuppression in most patients
B Is caused by an acid-fast coccobacillus
C Does not spread by the haematogenous route
D Has significant constitutional symptoms as a feature
E Is best treated by a one week course of high dose erythromycin

IN20 Mycoplasma pulmonary infections

A Are highly contagious

B Demonstrate intracellular inclusions in respiratory epithelial cells
C Are the commonest cause of the acute chest syndrome in patients with sickle cell disease
D Have a severity of illness which correlates with the titre of cold agglutinins
E Cause symptoms which are generally more severe than clinical signs would suggest

ANSWERS

IN1

A False — the classic cutaneous lesion of Lyme disease is erythema chronicum migrans, an annular rash with a clear central area

B True — the vector for the spirochete is a tick called *Ixodes danmii* whose most common host is the deer

C True

D False — children less than 8 years old should not be treated with tetracyclines; penicillin and erythromycin are acceptable alternatives

E True — there are various stages of disease. Stage 1 lasts 3–4 weeks and is characterised by lymphadenopathy, meningoencephalopathy and hepatosplenomegaly. Systemic upset is common with headaches and chills. The classic lesion of stage 1 disease is erythema chronicum migrans (in 85% of cases). Stage 2 disease may follow several weeks or months later in untreated cases. Meningitis and cranial nerve palsies and musculoskeletal problems occur. Cardiac abnormalities including heart block occur in 10%, usually within 5 weeks of the illness. Stage 3 disease can be a persistent erosive arthritis occasionally with intellectual impairment. The classic skin lesion in stage 3 disease is acrodermatitis chronica atrophicans

IN2

A True

B False — the rash is an erythroderma-like sunburn and varies from mild to severe

C True

D False — the fever is consistently high

E True — the host major histocompatibility antigens are expressed most highly in skin, gastrointestinal and liver cells, which are therefore the organs most affected by graft-versus-host disease. Chronic graft-versus-host disease is more like a multisystem disorder

IN3

A True

B False — it causes thrombocytopenia

C True — IgE and IgA are markedly elevated and IgM diminished
D True
E True

IN4

A True — this causes failure to kill phagocytosed catalase-positive organisms such as staphylococcus
B True — in 60% of cases
C True — this can be used to screen for polymorph function
D True — apart from superoxide generation polymorphonuclear function is normal
E True — CGD is clinically characterised by recurrent pyogenic infections in infancy. Pneumonias are common and lymphadenopathy almost universal

IN5

A False — this is an inactivated vaccine
B False — this is an inactivated vaccine
C False — this is also inactivated
D True — other live vaccines include oral polio, rubella and yellow fever
E True

IN6

A False — most cases occur between the ages of 6 and 18 months. It is rare after 3 years
B True
C True
D False — the child usually looks well despite the high temperature
E False — desquamation is rare

IN7

A False — it is an RNA virus in the family Paramyxoviridae, genus Morbillivirus
B False — it is very infectious and is rarely subclinical
C False — the airborne route is the most common mode of spread during an epidemic but spread by droplet spray from the respiratory tract and direct contact are important means of cross infection

D False — measles is infectious from the 10th day of incubation to the 4th day of the rash

E False — the rash starts as faint macules behind the ears and on the neck, cheeks and hairline, and is preceded by conjunctivitis and Koplick's spots in the mouth. It then spreads to the whole face, neck, upper arms and chest within 24 h, becoming more maculopapular. During the next 24 h it spreads to the back, abdomen and thighs

IN8

A True

B False — aminoglycosides or newer beta-lactamase-resistant penicillins are required to combat pseudomonas infections

C False — pseudomonas infection of sinuses is unusual

D True — pseudomonas infection of the respiratory tract is unusual in immunocompetent hosts. In cystic fibrosis patients it is excessive host response rather than active bacterial invasion that appears to cause the severe problems associated with pseudomonas colonisation

E True

IN9

A True — vaccine-induced measles antibody develops more rapidly than that following natural infection so MMR can be used to protect susceptible contacts during a measles outbreak.

B False — antibody response to the mumps and rubella components of MMR vaccine are too slow for effective prophylaxis after exposure to these infections

C True — this occurs in about 1% of children up to 4 years

D False — it should be given irrespective of a history of measles, mumps or rubella infection or measles immunisation

E True — other contraindications include children presenting for vaccination with a significant febrile illness, those who have received another live vaccine within three weeks and those with allergies to neomycin or kanamycin

IN10

A True

B True — second trimester infection may cause miscarriage and in the third trimester may lead to preterm labour

C True

D False — it is usually contracted from contaminated foods especially coleslaw, soft cheeses and processed chicken

E False — ampicillin plus gentamicin is often used as treatment

IN11

A True

B True — this may be caused by *Neisseria gonorrhoea* or *Chlamydia trachomatis* infections

C False

D False

E True — mumps, measles and rubella are notifiable

IN12

A False — these do not occur despite recurrent severe infections

B True

C False — IgM levels are virtually undetectable

D True — progressive pulmonary damage may result from infections, typically with common organisms such as haemophilus, staphylococcus and streptococcus

E True — one form is X-linked Bruton's disease but presentation of other forms may be delayed with chronic sinusitis being a problem in these cases

IN13

A True — the other features are X-linked inheritance and eczema

B False — the associations of Di George syndrome include heart disease, especially conotruncal disorders, urinary tract anomalies and abnormal facies

C True — Bruton's agammaglobulinaemia patients may suffer recurrent septic arthritis

D True — IgA is the major immunoglobulin of the respiratory and gastrointestinal tracts

E True — both T and B cell function are deficient. A matched donor transplant may provide a longlasting cure

IN14

A False — it is due to *Vibrio cholerae*, a Gram-negative rod

B False — contaminated water and food, especialy shellfish, play a major role in transmission

C False — the site of infection is the small intestine

D False — the incubation period is 6 hours to 5 days

E False — the vaccine does not reduce the rate of unapparent infections and is therefore not useful in preventing transmission of cholera within families or communities

IN15

A False — *Staphylococcus aureus* is responsible for 90% of cases in the absence of intravenous lines or catheters

B False — staphylococci are common commensals and not all types are invasive

C True

D True — especially influenza

E False — cooked food stored at greater than 7°C causes two-thirds of cases. Illness usually follows within 4 h of ingestion of an enterotoxigenic strain of *Staphylococcus aureus*. Coagulase-negative staphylococcal food poisoning is much less common

IN16

A True — this is an area of reduced phagocytosis and relatively stagnant blood flow

B False — older children's joints are protected by a more definite growth plate. Young children have blood vessels that bridge the physeal area and their joints are more vulnerable

C True

D True — in untreated cases the ESR and C-reactive protein are raised in 80–90% of cases

E True — discitis is usually a differential diagnosis in children under 5 years in whom the disc is still well vascularised

IN17

A False — hepatosplenomegaly, lymphadenopathy, recurrent candidias and diarrhoea can appear in the first months but rarely in the neonatal period

B False — infants should be immunised at the normal times

C False — the Salk killed polio vaccine should be substituted for the oral polio vaccine

D True

E False — there is a fall in the ratio of helper to suppressor cells

IN18

A True

B True — however the MMR vaccine has drastically reduced the overall incidence

C True — polymerase chain reaction (PCR) tests may detect measles RNA

D False — the children have usually made a full recovery from an 'ordinary' measles illness before developing SSPE 7–10 years later

E False — the M matrix protein is usually absent. IgG and IgM raised against other particles may be found. An oligoclonal rise in CSF immunoglobins may be found

IN19

A True

B True — it is caused by weakly acid-fast Gram-positive aerobes

C False — it is spread by the haematogenous route, usually from a primary lung infection, causing multisystem disease

D True

E False — sulphonamides or imipenem and amikacin should be used for a minimum of six weeks. Surgical treatment of abscesses may be required.

IN20

A False — they are not highly communicable so families become infected slowly

B False — mycoplasma are the smallest free-living organisms

C True

D True

E True

10: Metabolic Disorders

*Answers to this section are to be found
between pages 89 and 92*

QUESTIONS

MN1 Hurler's syndrome
A Is due to a defect of idurosulphate sulphatase
B Is X-linked
C Presents at birth with cloudy corneas
D Is distinguished from the other mucopolysaccharidoses by the excretion of dermatan sulphate in the urine
E Results in 'gargoyle' cells

MN2 In the lipidoses
A Krabbe's disease is associated with globoid histiocytes
B Niemann–Pick disease is associated with foamy histiocytes
C Diffuse angiokeratomosis occurs in Fabry's disease
D Patients with Gm1 gangliosidosis have a profound deficiency of acid beta-galactosidase activity in their leukocytes
E Gaucher's disease is due to a deficiency of hexosaminidase

MN3 Hypertriglyceridaemia occurs in children with
A Diabetes mellitus
B Hyperthyroidism
C Type 1 glycogen storage disease
D Anorexia nervosa
E Nephrotic syndrome

MN4 In disorders of the urea cycle
A Acidosis and raised ammonia levels are characteristic
B The incidence is 1 in 1000 live births
C Ornithine transcarbamylase (OTC) deficiency may be distinguished from transient hyperammonaemia of the newborn by the finding of high urinary orotic acid levels
D Maternal carriers of OTC may have a forme fruste of the disease
E Arginine replacement therapy is ineffective

85

MN5 Lesch–Nyhan syndrome

A Leads to destructive behaviour due to inability to feel pain
B Is inherited as an autosomal recessive condition
C Is due to hypoxanthine guanine phosphoribosyl transferase deficiency
D Leads to a marked increase in the urinary excretion of uric acid
E Is due to a defect in the 'purine salvage' pathway

MN6 Niemann–Pick disease

A Is inherited as an autosomal dominant disease
B Has characteristic appearances on bone marrow aspirate
C Is associated with a cherry red spot on the optic disc in 50% of cases
D Has benign forms
E Is associated with failure to reach early milestones at the correct time

MN7 Lactic acidosis

A Is characterized by deep sighing respirations of the Kussmaul variety
B Occurs in galactosaemia
C Occurs in carnitine deficiency syndrome
D Occurs in Leigh subacute necrotizing encephalopathy
E Occurs in thiamine deficiency

MN8 Acute intermittent porphyria

A Is inherited in an autosomal dominant pattern
B May present as appendicitis
C May be suggested by abnormal urinary metabolites even between attacks
D Is characterized by diarrhoea
E Is not associated with cutaneous changes

MN9 In Graves' disease

A There is peripheral lymphocytosis
B There are an equal number of affected males and females
C Osseous development is delayed for age
D Splenomegaly occurs
E Craniostenosis occurs

MN10 In phenylketonuria

A There is tyrosine hydroxylase deficiency
B Clincal signs and symptoms first occur in puberty
C Affected individuals usually have brown hair and brown eyes
D There is a characteristic odour of must
E If a low phenylalanine diet is not adhered to in pregnancy there is an increased incidence of congenital heart disease in children

MN11 Diabetic ketoacidosis

A Requires replacement of estimated fluid deficit over 4–8 h
B Is outruled by normal glucose levels
C Is associated with signs of cerebral oedema at presentation
D May be associated with hyperkalaemia despite increased losses
E Is treated with a loading dose of insulin 0.01 i.u./kg intravenously

MN12 Albinism

A Which is oculocutaneous is inherited in an autosomal dominant manner
B Which is partial is inherited in an autosomal recessive manner
C Of the ocular type causes nystagmus
D In the partial form must be differentiated from Waardenburg syndrome
E Occurs in all races

MN13 Hyperammonaemia

A Due to a urea cycle defect is commonly associated with neutropenia
B May be treated with sodium benzoate
C Occurs as a transient phenomenon in the newborn
D Treatment includes peritoneal dialysis
E Is associated with a high level of blood urea nitrogen

MN14 Pompes disease

A Is a type 2 glycogen storage disease
B Is due to acid maltase deficiency
C Is characterized by multiple joint contractures
D Is inherited in an autosomal recessive fashion
E Results in an enlarged tongue with fasciculations

MN15 Hypoparathyroidism

A Occurs secondary to hypomagnesaemia
B Is part of Di George syndrome
C Results in shortened Q–T interval
D Treatment includes a vitamin D analogue
E Is associated with renal stones

ANSWERS

MN1

A False — this deficiency causes Hunter's syndrome (mucopolysaccharidosis type 2). Hurler's syndrome is caused by a deficiency of alpha-L-iduronidase. This causes increased urinary and tissue levels of heparin and dermatan.

B False — it is an autosomal recessive disease

C False — infants appear normal at birth. Signs of organomegaly, kyphosis and coarsening of facies develop progressively

D False — only enzyme assays are definitive

E True — these are mucopolysaccharide-laden lysosomes

MN2

A True — the enzyme deficiency is beta-galactosidase

B True

C True — this is an X-linked recessive disorder

D True — the phenotype may be very similar to Hurler's syndrome

E False — the enzyme deficiency is of beta-glucososidase

MN3

A True

B False — hypothyroidism causes raised cholesterol and triglyceride levels

C True

D False — obesity is the commonest cause of raised triglycerides

E True — protein loss in the urine causes compensatory increased hepatic synthesis and therefore raised lipoprotein levels. Serum lipoprotein lipase levels are also reduced

MN4

A False — acidosis is a feature of organic acidaemias

B False — it is much rarer, approximately 1 in 30 000–50 000 live births

C True

D True

E False — arginine replacement is beneficial as it supplies ornithine and N-acetyl glutamate. It is not effective in organic acidaemias

MN5

A False — the children compulsively self harm but can feel pain
B False — it is X-linked and would be expected to be seen in males only, although recently some female patients have been described
C True
D True
E True

MN6

A False — like most enzyme deficiency syndromes it is autosomal recessive
B True — cells are characteristically foam laden
C False — the cherry red spot is on the macula
D True — type B has few neurological manifestations and has a normal lifespan. Types C and D have normal sphingomyelinase levels
E True — the achievement of milestones may be delayed but they are reached. Failure to thrive and feeding difficulties predominate the early presentation at 3–5 months

MN7

A True
B False — acidosis is not a feature of classical galactosaemia
C True — presentation can be with fasting hypoglycaemia in the first year of life or more commonly with progressive cardiac and skeletal myopathy in the first 2–5 years
D True — other features are psychomotor retardation, optic atrophy and hypotonia
E True

MN8

A True
B True — porphyrias can present in several ways and an acute abdomen with abnormally coloured urine should prompt further investigations
C False — abnormal urinary metabolites are only found during attacks
D False — constipation may be a feature
E True

MN9

A True — Graves' thyrotoxicosis is immune mediated and a lympho-cytosis may be found

B False — female patients outnumber males by approximately 10 : 1

C False — thyroxine advances bone age

D True — generalised lymphadenopathy may also be found

E True

MN10

A False — the deficiency is of phenylalanine hydroxylase leading to excessive accumulation of phenylalanine

B False — untreated infants show developmental delay before 1 year of age

C False — blonde hair and blue eyes are characteristic

D True

E True — microcephaly is also more common. Females need careful counselling and adequate family planning advice

MN11

A False — therapy aims to restore deficiency over 24–48 h. Overra-pid correction has been linked to 'coning' from cerebral oedema

B False — a normal glucose level does not exclude acidosis and the serum bicarbonate must be measured

C False — these signs may develop in the second 12–24 h

D True — total body potassium may be depleted despite normal or increased plasma levels

E False — the dose is 0.1 i.u./kg intravenously

MN12

A False — it is inherited in an autosomal recessive fashion

B False — it is inherited in an autosomal dominant manner

C True — and there is also reduced visual acuity

D True — those with Waardenburg syndrome have a white forelock, heterochromia and hearing impairment

E True

MN13

A False

B True — this allows excretion of NH_3 in the form of hippurate

C True — the levels are rarely greater than 150 μmol/l

D True — ammonia is easily dialysable and *in utero* placental dialysis prevents accumulation before birth

E False — the levels are usually low

MN14

A False — it is a type 3 glycogen storage disease

B True — this is the debranching enzyme with facilitates mobilisation of glycogen

C False — joint contractures are rare

D True

E True — cardiac and muscle involvement may be prominent

MN15

A True — post-neonatal onset of hypoparathyroidism may be idiopathic or secondary to irradiation, neck surgery, haemosiderosis or hypomagnesaemia

B True — this syndrome consists of immunodeficiency, hypoparathyroidism, congenital heart defects and abnormal facies

C False — the Q–T interval is prolonged

D True — oral calcium supplements and a vitamin D analogue are used for treatment. Acute hypocalcaemia is treated with intravenous 10% calcium gluconate

E False — the clinical signs and symptoms are due to hypocalcaemia which results from decreased renal calcium reabsorption and bone resorption

11: Neonatology

*Answers to this section are to be found
between pages 97 and 100*

QUESTIONS

N1 The following are correct regarding intraventricular haemorrhage
A The germinal matrix is most prominent after the 28th week of gestation
B Grade 1–2 intraventricular haemorrhage (IVH) has little effect on neurodevelopmental outcome
C Grade 3 haemorrhage incudes parenchymal haemorrhage
D Post-haemorrhagic ventricular dilatation (+ or – hydrocephalus) independently adversely affects neurodevelopmental outcome
E Post-haemorrhagic ventricular dilatation spontaneously arrests or resolves in 10% of cases

N2 The following are associated with a large anterior fontanelle
A Intrauterine growth retardation
B Osteogenesis imperfecta
C Apert's syndrome
D Hypophosphatasia
E William's syndrome

N3 ABO incompatibility is suggested by
A Fetal hydrops
B Parental consanguinity
C A blood film showing megaloblastosis
D Maternal blood group A
E Severe early jaundice

N4 The following conditions are associated with polyhydramnios
A Encephalocele
B Renal dysplasia
C Achondroplasia
D Trisomy 21
E Maternal diabetes mellitus

N5 Congenital syphilis
A May cause splenomegaly
B Is associated with choanal stenosis
C Should provoke CSF examination
D Is associated with high placental weight
E Causes a maculopapular rash

N6 In congenital hypothyroidism
A The diagnosis is suggested by absent epiphyses on knee X-ray in a full-term infant
B Propranolol is the treatment of choice
C The diagnosis may be made from a routine screening test in the newborn period
D Late features include poor feeding and constipation
E Therapy is rarely needed beyond 3 months of age

N7 A baby born to a hepatitis B surface antigen (H BsAg) positive mother
A Is infectious to staff handling body fluids
B That receives hep B vaccine and immune globulin should have its DPT and Hib vaccines delayed 1 month
C Should not be breast fed
D Is at higher risk of infection if e antigen is present in the mother
E Is more likely to become a carrier if of Chinese origin

N8 The following conditions cause respiratory distress
A Wilson–Mikity syndrome
B Polycythaemia
C Myotonic dystrophy
D Turner's syndrome
E Potter sequence

N9 Conjugated hyperbilirubinaemia occurs in
A Crigler–Najjar syndrome
B Breast feeding
C Dubin–Johnson syndrome
D Choledochal cyst
E Tyrosinosis

N10 In multiple gestation pregnancies

A Twin–twin transfusion may have occurred if the haemoglobin differs by more than 5 g/l

B Monoaminotic twins have the lowest mortality rate

C Oesophageal atresia is more common than in singleton births

D Placental and vascular anomalies are more common

E Monozygotic twins are more common in Caucasians than other races

N11 Causes of hypokalaemia in the neonate include

A Congenital adrenal hyperplasia

B Hyperaldosteronism

C Acute renal failure

D Alkalosis

E Diuretic therapy

N12 Infants of drug abusing mothers

A Are 100 times more likely to suffer a sudden infant death

B Are more likely to be anaemic

C Who abused methadone are more likely to suffer severe neonatal jaundice

D May have disturbed thyroid hormone levels

E Who have severe withdrawal symptoms usually do so 6–8 h following delivery

N13 The following clinical features occur in neonatal polycythaemia

A Hyperglycaemia

B Jaundice

C Respiratory distress

D Hypotonia

E Thrombocytopenia

N14 A patent ductus arteriosus

A Usually closes functionally within 1–2 h of birth

B That is large may result in Eisenmenger syndrome

C Closes following a prostaglandin infusion

D Persists in pulmonary atresia due to arterial hypoxaemia

E That is small produces a continuous murmur in the pulmonary area below the left clavicle

N15 Microcephaly
A Is usually a genetically inherited condition
B Is defined as a head circumference more than three standard deviations below the mean for age and sex
C Occurs in fetal alcohol syndrome
D Occurs following intrauterine infections
E Occurs in neurofibromatosis

ANSWERS

N1

A False — the germinal matrix is the tissue of origin of the sub-ependymal blood vessels implicated in the origin of IVH. It is most prominent between 24 and 28 weeks

B True — unless associated with parenchymal ischaemia or haemorrhage the outlook is good

C False — grade 1 is subependymal bleeding, grade 2 involves intraventricular haemorrhage without dilatation, grade 3 is dilatation of ventricles by haemorrhage and grade 4 is parenchymal haemorrhage

D False — more than half of the cases resolve

E False — it arrests or resolves in more than 50% of cases, if it is progressive and requires shunting or repeated CSF taps the prognosis is poor

N2

A True

B True

C True

D True

E False

N3

A False — the condition is usually mild and rarely leads to intrauterine problems

B False — diagnosis may be difficult as the direct Coombs' test may be negative. It may be confirmed by detecting anti-A or anti-B IgG in the mother's plasma and detecting this antibody on the baby's red cells

C False

D False — infants are usually A (or more rarely B) and mother's blood group O

E False — most infants with ABO incompatibility have only mild or moderate early jaundice

N4

A True

B False — this may cause oligohydramnios

C True

D True — 5% of cases of polyhydramnios have an underlying chromosomal abnormality. The greater the polyhydramnios the greater the risk of abnormality

E True

N5

A True

B False — infants may get a blood-stained nasal discharge, not associated with choanal stenosis

C True — the CSF may be abnormal even in the absence of clinical signs of meningitis

D True — congenital syphilis is a cause of hydrops fetalis which causes the placenta to be larger than normal

E True

N6

A True

B False — propranolol is part of the treatment of hyperthyroidism

C True — although serum levels of T3, T4 and TSH must be measured for confirmation

D True — the classic features of cretinism are also absent at birth

E False — treatment is life-long unless the hypothyroidism is due to a transient problem such as maternal anti-thyroid medication

N7

A True — this is especially so if the mother is e antigen positive

B False — there is no reason to delay routine immunisations

C False — this is not a contraindication to breast feeding

D True

E True — 40–70% of infants of Chinese mothers become carriers compared to 30% of those born to African mothers and 10% of Indian mothers

N8

A True — these infants develop oxygen dependence in the 2nd or 3rd week of life

B True

C True — this is due to neuromuscular dysfunction and has a poor prognosis
D False
E True — there is pulmonary hypoplasia

N9
A False — this causes unconjugated hyperbilirubinaemia
B False — this causes unconjugated hyperbilirubinaemia
C True
D True — this may cause biliary obstruction
E True

N10
A True — the baby who receives the transfusion is more at risk from polycythaemia than the other infant is from anaemia
B False — they have the highest mortality rate
C True
D True
E False — the rate of monozygotic twinning is unaffected by race

N11
A False — this classically causes hyponatraemia and hyperkalaemia
B True
C False — this is a cause of hyperkalaemia
D True
E True

N12
A False — the incidence of sudden infant death is 10 times the normal rate
B True
C True
D True — their irritability is due to drug withdrawal rather than altered thyroid function
E False — severe withdrawal reactions begin 24–48 h after birth and may persist for several weeks

N13
A False — hypoglycaemia may be found in a polycythaemic baby

Neonatology

B True
C True
D True
E True

Babies at risk of polycythaemia include preterm small-for-gestational age infants, infants of diabetic mothers, twin–twin transfusions or cases of simple delay of clamping of the cord

N14

A False — it normally closes functionally within 10–15 h of birth
B True — this is the reversal of a left to right shunt because of the development of pulmonary hypertension
C False — prostaglandins maintain patency
D True — this supports pulmonary circulation until corrective surgery can be performed
E True — the heart is of normal size and the pulses and blood pressure normal. The classic continuous murmur is heard in the pulmonary area below the clavicle and becomes louder in the horizontal position unlike the venous hum which disappears in the horizontal position

N15

A False — microcephaly is often of unknown aetiology but is associated with certain chromosome defects such as trisomies 9, 13 and 22
B True
C True
D True — it is a typical feature of the congenital rubella syndrome
E False — a large head circumference would be a more typical finding

12: Neurology

Answers to this section are to be found
between pages 106 and 111

QUESTIONS

NU1 Febrile convulsions

A Frequently occur in neonates
B Are inherited in an autosomal dominant fashion
C That recur in subsequent infections should be treated with anticonvulsants
D Usually occur in the early stages of illness
E Should prompt lumbar puncture in most cases

NU2 In myasthenia gravis

A Pupillary responses to light are preserved
B Infants that are transiently affected by maternal antibodies are at increased risk of developing myasthenia gravis later in childhood
C Muscle biopsy may show an inflammatory infiltrate
D Infants should not undergo edrophonium testing
E Thymectomy is ineffective in familial forms

NU3 Benign intracranial hypertension

A Is also known as pseudotumour cerebri
B Is associated with otitis media
C Usually presents as sudden visual loss
D Occurs as a complication of long-term oral tetracycline treatment
E Is usually self-limiting without sequelae

NU4 In neurofibromatosis type 1

A Bilateral acoustic neuromata are a feature
B Precocious sexual development may occur
C Visual acuity is severely reduced if optic gliomas are present
D Complex partial seizures are a common complication
E Diagnosis requires the presence of two plexiform neuroma

NU5 In hydrocephalus

A In the Dandy–Walker malformation there is a developmental failure of the fourth ventricle
B Separation of the cranial sutures leads to the 'crack-pot' sign
C In infants the eyes appear deviated upwards
D Spasticity and ataxia affect the arms more than the legs
E Of late childhood there may be no appreciable enlargement of the head

NU6 Krabbe's disease

A Is characterised by Schwann cell hypertrophy
B Is caused by beta-galactosidase deficiency
B May present as colic
D Occurs only in males
E Of late onset disease is often characterised by ataxia

NU7 In Guillain–Barré syndrome

A Females are affected more often than males
B Sensory symptoms are more striking than paralysis
C Muscle wasting is usual
D Cranial nerve involvement is common
E Sinus tachycardia is common in the acute phase

NU8 In Retts syndrome

A The male : female incidence ratio is 2 : 1
B Early milestones are achieved normally
C An abnormal respiratory pattern may emerge
D Hydrocephalus is common
E Dystonic postures are an early feature

NU9 In Gilles de la Tourette's syndrome

A The symptoms disappear completely in sleep
B Abnormal vocalisation is common as the initial symptom
C There is a greater prevalence in Japan than the UK
D Average survival is 10–15 years
E Haloperidol reduces symptoms in the majority of patients

NU10 In common migraine in children

A An aura occurs

B There is intense nausea and vomiting

C Vitamin A is useful for prophylaxis

D Paternal history of migraine is more frequent than maternal history

E The presentation may be confused with porphyria cutanea tarda

NU11 Communicating hydrocephalus is caused by

A Aqueductal stenosis

B Arnold–Chiari malformation

C Pneumococcal meningitis

D Achondroplasia

E Dandy–Walker malformation

NU12 In tuberose sclerosis (TS)

A The EEG may show hypsarrhythymia

B ACTH therapy leads to an improvement in the EEG

C Retinal phakomata cause visual disturbances

D Axillary freckling is a feature

E Cardiac rhabdomyomata are more common in adults than children

NU13 Benign intracranial hypertension

A Is associated with abnormalities of vitamin A metabolism

B Presents more frequently with vomiting than is the case with brain tumours

C Causes focal neurological signs

D May result from brain tumours

E Does not affect the size of the blind spot

NU14 With regard to brain tumours

A Astrocytomas are usually sited in the posterior fossa in children

B Medullablastomas are more often seen in adolescents than in younger children

C Ependymomas are the most common brain tumours in childhood

D Craniopharyngiomas develop from squamous cell rests in Rathke's pouch

E The diencephalic syndrome may result from tumours in the hypothalamic region

NU15 Neurological deterioration occurs in association with
A Glycogen storage disease type 2
B Non-ketotic hyperglycinaemia
C Tyrosinaemia type 1
D Maple syrup urine disease
E Absence seizures

NU16 Optic neuritis in childhood
A Is characterised by gradual deterioration in vision
B May be secondary to cytotoxic therapy
C May be associated with painful eye movements
D Is rarely an isolated finding
E May show myelinated nerve fibres on fundoscopy

NU17 Megalencephaly occurs in
A Tay–Sachs disease
B Absence of corpus callosum
C Phenytoin fetopathy
D A familial form
E Tuberose sclerosis

NU18 In Charcot–Marie–Tooth disease (hereditary sensorimotor neuropathy type 1)
A Inheritance may be autosomal dominant or recessive
B Progressive weakness of ankle dorsiflexion is characteristic
C Proprioceptive sensation is preserved
D Nerve conduction velocities are reduced
E Pupillary responses are normal

NU19 Simple absence seizures
A Often have an aura
B Do not have a post-ictal state
C Have an equal sex incidence
D May be associated with automatic behaviour
E Are produced by breath holding

NU20 Hypsarrhythmia on an EEG trace
A Is seen in tuberose sclerosis

B Is seen in untreated phenylketonuria (PKU)
C Is associated with infantile spasms
D Usually appears around six weeks of age
E May be enhanced by sleep

ANSWERS

NU1

A False — febrile fits almost never occur in children under 6 months of age. Fits which occur in this age group need investigating. The peak incidence of febrile convulsions is at 18–20 months of age

B False — there is a familial tendency but no inheritance pattern has been identified

C False — there is no benefit from prophylactic anticonvulsants in uncomplicated cases

D True

E False — they are related to the degree of fever and not the location of the infection. Lumbar puncture may be necessary in younger children without an obvious focus of infection. These children may not display the classic signs of meningitis

NU2

A True

B False — transient neonatal myasthenia gravis needs to be distinguished from a rare, hereditary congenital myasthenia gravis

C True — inflammatory changes may occur; these are referred to as lymphorrhages

D True — edrophonium may cause cardiac arrhythmias in young infants

E True

NU3

A True

B True

C False — sixth nerve palsy and an enlarged blind spot are common but sudden visual loss is rare. Headache is invariably present and nausea and vomiting occur

D True — other causes include trauma and infections

E True — it is largely a self-limiting condition although repeated lumbar punctures, steroids and acetazolamide may sometimes be used in the management of this condition

NU4

A False — acoustic neuromata occur in neurofibromatosis type 2, which accounts for 10% of all cases of neurofibromatosis

B True — this is secondary to tumour invasion or compression of the hypothalamus

C False — optic gliomas are present in 15% and most are asymptomatic and have normal or near-normal vision

D True

E False — neurofibromatosis type 1 is diagnosed if any 2 of the following signs are present: axillary or inguinal freckling, two or more iris Lisch nodules, a distinctive osseous lesion, at least five *café-au-lait* spots greater than 5 mm in diameter in prepubertal individuals, two or more neurofibromas or one plexiform neurofibroma, optic glioma, or a first degree relative with neurofibromatosis type 1

NU5

A True — this results in cystic expansion of the fourth ventricle and management involves shunting the cystic cavity

B True

C False — the eyes deviate downwards producing the 'setting sun' sign

D False — long tract signs are more common in the legs than the arms

E True — in the older child the cranial sutures are partially closed so signs of hydrocephalus may be more subtle

NU6

A False — this is a neurodegenerative disorder characterised by myelin loss and the presence of globoid bodies in the white matter

B True

C True — it usually presents in the first months of life with crying, irritability, vomiting, and feeding problems, often thought to be due to colic

D False — it occurs in both sexes and is inherited, like most enzyme defects, as an autosomal recessive disorder

E True — in late onset disease there may be progressive gait disturbances, with spasticity or ataxia

NU7

A False — there is a male : female ratio of between 2 : 1 and 3 : 2

B False — sensory symptoms are usually less striking than paralysis but in some cases painful parasthaesiae of the hands and feet are complained of before the onset of weakness

C False — muscles are often tender on palpation but not wasted

D True — the facial nerve is most frequently involved, often bilaterally

E True — cardiac arrythmias may also occur

NU8

A False — this is a neurodegenerative disorder occurring exclusively in females

B True — development proceeds normally until 1 year of age when regression of language and motor milestones occurs

C True — there may be abnormal sighing respirations with intermittent periods of apnoea

D False — microcephaly occurs, not hydrocephalus

E False — an ataxic gait or fine tremor of the hands is an early neurologic finding

NU9

A True — symptoms disappear in sleep and are aggravated by anxiety

B False — abnormal vocalisation occurs in all cases but it is rarely the initial symptom

C True — it is more common in Japan and the USA than in the UK

D False — it is not a progressive disorder so prognosis for survival is very good, but the prognosis for recovery is not good

E True — haloperidol abolishes or reduces symptoms in 80–90% of cases

NU10

A False — common migraine is the most prevalent type of migraine in childhood and there is no aura. A visual aura precedes the headache in classic migraine

B True — this is a characteristic feature

C False — drugs used for prophylaxis include propranolol and phenytoin. Methysergide and amitriptyline are used for prophlaxis but not in young children

D False — a family history is present in 90% of cases but it is usually on the maternal side

E False — acute intermittent porphyria may present in a similar fashion to migraine

NU11

A False

B True

C True

D True

E False

NU12

A True — TS may present as infantile spasms. All such children should have a Wood's light examination for ash-leaf patches

B True

C False — they do not usually interfere with vision

D False — this is Crowe's sign, a feature of neurofibromatosis

E False — about 50% of children with TS have rhabdomyomata which tend to slowly resolve spontaneously

NU13

A True — hypervitaminosis A can cause benign intracranial hypertension

B False

C False — although diplopia is common secondary to benign intracranial hypertension, focal signs suggest a space-occupying lesion or demyelination

D True — possibly due to venous obstruction. Other possible causes include sagittal sinus thrombosis, galactosaemia, hypothyroidism and tetracyline or oral contraceptive therapy

E False — after infancy, the most common findings are an increased blind spot and papilloedema

NU14

A True — they have a good prognosis

B False — medullablastomas are the most common brain tumour in children under 7 years of age. Supratentorial lesions predominate in adolescents as in adults

C False — they account for only 10% of posterior fossa tumours in childhood. Posterior fossa tumours account for 60% of tumours between the ages of 2 and 12 years

D True — 90% are visible as areas of calcification on skull X-ray or CT scan

E True — these children are grossly emaciated but usually cheerful as compared to children with coeliac disease or those who have been neglected

NU15

A False — neurological development is usually normal

B True — this fatal disease presents with progressive coma, lethargy and fitting around the third day of life. Few infants survive the first year

C False — untreated cases die of hepatic failure or in chronic cases hepatoma

D True — these children with the characteristic odour become more and more lethargic in the first week of life. Opisthotonus and hypoglycaemia are features but the neurological state does not improve with correction of hypoglycaemia. The long-term prognosis even in treated cases is poor

E False — neurological deterioration does not occur

NU16

A False — due to its inflammatory nature visual loss is usually acute and may be painful

B True — vincristine may cause optic neuritis as well as more typically symmetric distal peripheral neuropathy

C True

D True — encephalitis, multiple sclerosis and juvenile demyelinating diseases should be ruled out if possible

E False — demyelination is a feature. Myelinated nerve fibres are a normal variant

NU17

A True — megalencephaly means abnormally large brain whereas macrocephaly means large head. The term can also be applied to heavy brains with additional structural anomalies such as absence of the corpus callosum

B True

C False — this causes microcephaly

D True — there is a benign familial condition causing megalen-cephaly which is dominantly inherited

E True — also in neurofibromatosis

NU18

A True

B True — most people remain ambulatory despite progressive neuro-pathic changes

C False — large myelinated fibres conveying proprioceptive informa-tion may be affected. Parasthaesiae may also occur

D True — they are greatly reduced

E True — cranial nerves are spared

NU19

A False — they are not associated with an aura

B True

C False — they are more common in girls

D True — this is a frequent occurrence

E False — they may be produced by hyperventilation

NU20

A True

B True

C True

D False — it usually appears around 6 months of age and is rare before 3 months

E True — sleep records are important for assessment and monitoring response to treatment

13: Psychiatry and Social Medicine

Answers to this section are to be found
between pages 115 and 117

QUESTIONS

P1 Recognised features of anorexia nervosa include
A Hypokalaemia
B Loss of body hair
C Low levels of growth hormone
D Distant parenting
E Large family size

P2 Night terrors
A Usually begin in teenage years
B Are accompanied by signs of intense autonomic activity
C Occur during rapid eye movement (REM) sleep
D Have a strong family history
E Are usually self-limiting

P3 The following occur in bulimia nervosa
A Decreased Q–T interval on ECG
B Wandering atrial pacemaker
C Mediastinal emphysema
D Swelling of the parotid gland
E Erosion of dental enamel

P4 Cocaine
A Is derived from the coca plant
B Has a half-life of 4–8 h
C In high doses produces effects similar to those of amphetamines
D In the form of 'crack' is inhaled nasally
E Intoxication produces tachycardia and hypertension

P5 School refusal
A Is more common in children from social classes 1, 2 and 3
B Is more common in small families

C Is more common in girls
D Has a better prognosis than truancy
E Is the cause of 20% of cases of school non-attendance

P6 Children with hyperkinetic syndrome

A Are often quiet, passive children
B Have a peak of hyperactivity between 3 and 8 years
C Are commonly boys
D Benefit from treatment with stimulant drugs in some cases
E Have features which overlap with children with attention deficit disorders

P7 In Asperger's syndrome

A There is typically an immediate impression of clumsiness
B Imaginative symbolic play is limited
C The diagnosis is usually made around 18 months of age
D Children may do well at school academically
E Diagnosis may be made on neurophysical testing

P8 Nocturnal enuresis

A Is more common in girls
B Occurs in 5–10% of 10 year olds
C Usually represents a more serious problem then diurnal enuresis
D Should be investigated by DMSA renal isotope scan
E Usually responds to treatment with potassium citrate

P9 In cases of physical abuse of children

A The perpetrator is more likely to be an older sibling than an unrelated adult
B It is difficult to distinguish rib fractures caused by assault from those caused by cardiopulmonary resuscitation
C Torn epiphyses result from a swinging injury
D Retinal haemmorhages suggest asphyxiation
E Twenty per cent of siblings show evidence of physical abuse

P10 Autistic children

A Who are going to acquire useful speech have usually done so by 5 years of age
B Are usually girls

C Often use peripheral vision rather than central vision
D Should be treated with fenfluramine
E Often have no fear of danger

ANSWERS

P1

A True — alkalosis may also result from the bouts of vomiting

B False — lanugo hair is a typical feature

C False — growth hormone levels are typically raised. Levels of thyroid stimulating hormone are also raised. Diurnal variation of cortisol secretion is lost

D False — overclose parenting is thought to be an important factor

E False — there is an overrepresentation of intelligent children in small families whose parents have high expectations of them. Eating may be the only area in the child's life where she or he can express autonomy

P2

A False — the peak incidence is in 4–7-year-old boys

B True — the child appears terrified and remote from parental comforting manoeuvres

C False — they occur during stage 4 deep sleep

D True

E True

P3

A False — Q–T prolongation has been described in addition to findings of low voltage and S–T segment changes

B True — supraventricular tachycardias may be exacerbated by electrolyte abnormalities

C True — this may result from oesophageal rupture by forced vomiting

D True — this may suggest malnutrition

E True — this is due to the acidity of the vomitus

P4

A True

B False — its short half-life of ½–1 h means that repeated doses are often taken at short intervals

C True — tachycardia, sweating, dilated pupils and feelings of paranoia may be demonstrated

D False — crack is a cocaine base taken by inhalation of its smoke, usually from a pipe

E True

P5

A True

B True — separation anxiety appears to be at the root of the problem for both the child and the parent

C False

D True — the children are usually bright and eventually do well at school. School refusal is usually experienced at starting school, new terms or changes of school

E False — most school refusers behave well at school after they have settled in

P6

A False — they have a short attention span, are impulsive and overactive. They often interfere with other children's work and disrupt classroom routine

B True

C True — three times as many boys as girls are affected

D True — amphetamines have been used with success, largely based on American experiences

E True

P7

A True

B True — these children are thought to be of normal intelligence but lack social and interactive skills. They tend to play on their own with little or no imaginative play

C False — diagnosis is often delayed until school age although speech may be noted to be delayed

D True

E False — it is a clinical diagnosis although other conditions may need to be ruled out on neurophysical testing

P8

A False — boys are more commonly affected

B True — 10–20% of 5 year olds wet at night and 1% of adult males are enuretic

C False — nocturnal enuresis is very common and usually self-limiting. Persistent daytime wetting may suggest an underlying neurological or urological abnormality

D False — the diagnosis is usually made from the history

E False — alkalinisation of the urine makes little difference. Behavioural therapies are usual, although short-term relief may be achieved with desmopressin analogues taken intranasally or orally

P9

A False — siblings account for only 1% of perpetrators

B False — resuscitation rarely causes rib fractures in children

C True

D False — they are more commonly caused by shaking. Petechiae may suggest asphyxiation

E True — about 3% of children die from their injuries

P10

A True

B False — autism is four times more common in males

C True — they often concentrate on things at the periphery of their visual field and they often appear to 'look past' things

D False — drug treatments generally offer little benefit. Practical help on managing the child's behaviour should be offered to the parents

E True — they may have no fear of true dangers but develop fear of totally harmless things

14: Renal Medicine

Answers to this section are to be found between pages 122 and 126

QUESTIONS

RM1 Proximal renal tubular acidosis
A Results from a defect in proximal tubular resorption of bicarbonate
B Is characterised by hypercalcuria
C May be treated with oral sodium citrate
D Is also known as type 1 renal tubular acidosis
E Leads to progressive renal failure

RM2 In chronic renal failure
A Body growth is maintained until glomerular filtration rate falls to below 10% of normal
B Replacement of fat-soluble vitamins is necessary
C Calcium carbonate is an effective phosphate binder
D Secondary hyperparathyroidism may result from failure of renal 1 hydroxylation of vitamin D
E Eggs and milk are good safe sources of usable proteins

RM3 In Lowe's syndrome (oculocerebrorenal dystrophy)
A Development is normal
B Fanconi's syndrome occurs
C Hypertonia occurs
D There is frontal bossing
E There is frequently a history of visual problems on the father's side of the family

RM4 In nephrogenic diabetes insipidus
A Inheritance is autosomal recessive
B Infants prefer to drink water than milk
C There is retardation of skeletal maturation
D DDAVP (desmopressin) effects urine concentration
E Thiazide diuretics decrease free water clearance

RM5 In Bartter's syndrome

A Hyperkalaemia occurs
B Aldosterone levels are low
C Marked hypertension occurs
D Metabolic alkalosis is a feature
E Tetany may occur

RM6 In renal vein thrombosis

A Small kidneys are seen on ultrasound
B There is usually thrombocytopenia
C Contrast studies are the first line of investigation
D Anticoagulant therapy is of value
E The condition is usually unilateral

RM7 Urinary stones

A Occur in malignant disease
B May result from diuretic therapy
C May complicate Crohn's disease
D Due to cystinuria are best treated with oral acidification of urine
E Which are staghorn calculi are associated with proteus infections

RM8 In haemolytic uraemic syndrome

A There has been a decrease in incidence over the last 10 years
B Continuous heparin infusion therapy has benefit over conservative management
C Hypertension is usually more severe in infants and young children
D Prostacyclin activity is low
E Haemodialysis is preferable to peritoneal dialysis

RM9 In acute renal failure

A The commonest aetiology in infants and toddlers is haemolytic uraemic syndrome
B Carboplatin is less commonly implicated than cisplatin
C Fractional urinary excretion of sodium is usually less than 1% in cases of prerenal renal failure
D The earliest ECG sign of hyperkalaemia is shortening of the P–R interval
E Calcium gluconate infusion causes an average reduction of serum potassium of 1 mmol/l

RM10 Proteinuria

A Occurs in renal tubular acidosis
B Is accompanied by an increase in C3 complement level in orthostatic proteinuria
C Occurs in vitamin A intoxication
D Occurs as a transient phenomenon in pyrexial patients
E Of 'tubular' origin has albumin as a major protein

RM11 Vesicoureteric reflux

A Causes 50% of endstage renal failure in children
B Is facilitated by abnormal medial emplacement of the ureters into the bladder
C In a duplex system usually affects the lower ureter
D Is present in 50% of cases of neuropathic bladder
E Of grades 1 and 2 resolves spontaneously in 10% of cases

RM12 In congenital nephrotic syndrome

A There is dilatation of the proximal convoluted tubule
B The placenta is small with areas of infarction
C Proteinuria first becomes apparent at about 3 months of age
D Secondary causes include mercury intoxication
E The sex incidence is equal

RM13 In minimal change nephrotic syndrome

A The typical age of onset is 3 years
B Immunofluorescence studies are positive
C There is increased incidence in females
D Gross haematuria is characteristic
E There are low fibrinogen levels

RM14 Kidney malformations occur in

A Di George sequence
B Tuberose sclerosis
C Jeune thoracic dystrophy
D Distal arthrogryposis
E Beckwith–Wiedemann syndrome

RM15 The following may cause interstitial nephritis

A Thiazide diuretics

B Lithium
C Carbamazepine
D Rifampicin
E Ranitidine

ANSWERS

RM1

A True

B False — this is not a feature

C True — large quantities may be required, oral bicarbonate may also be used

D False — proximal renal tubular acidosis is type 2, distal renal tubular acidosis is type 1

E False — renal failure does not usually occur, in fact the condition may improve with age

RM2

A False — if the glomerular filtration rate falls below 50% the growth rate falls

B False — water-soluble vitamins may be deficient due to poor diet or loss in dialysis

C True

D True

E True — uraemia results from build-up of nitrogenous waste. Proteins from milk and eggs have high 'biological value' and metabolism into nitrogeneous products is minimal

RM3

A False — there is marked developmental delay

B True

C False — hypotonia is present with decreased or absent reflexes

D True — this is a feature along with cataracts, buphthalmos and cryptorchidism

E False — this condition is X-linked and the mother and other carrier females may have cataracts, aminoaciduria and mental retardation

RM4

A False — inheritance is usually X-linked recessive

B True — the deficit is of water rather than liquid *per se*

C True — there is failure to grow, and retarded skeletal and intellectual development

D False — the kidney is unresponsive to vasopressin and its analogues. A patient who responds to DDAVP by increasing urinary osmolality does not have nephrogenic diabetes insipidus

E True — this paradoxical response is due to total body depletion of sodium. The proximal tubule will consequently increase resorption of sodium and free water, so the distal tubule is presented with less water

RM5

A False — there is marked hypokalaemia

B False — serum aldosterone and renin levels are increased

C False — Bartter's syndrome may be difficult to distinguish from primary hyperaldosteronism due to an adrenal tumour but hypertension distinguishes the two as it does not occur in Bartter's syndrome

D True

E True — presentation may be with polyuria, polydypsia, poor weight gain, vomiting, weakness or tetany

RM6

A False — marked enlargement of the kidneys is seen on ultrasound

B True — this is due to platelet consumption in the thrombus

C False — they should be avoided to minimise risk of further renovascular damage

D False — treatment involves correction of fluid and electrolyte abnormalities, and treatment of infection

E True — bilateral involvement results in acute renal failure

RM7

A True — stones form due to high tissue turnover and consequent high purine levels causing stones

B True

C True — due to failure of enteropathic circulation of bile acids leading to excessive colonic reabsorption of oxalate and hence to oxaluria

D False — the urine should be alkalinised to increase solubility of cystine

E True — alkaline urine is more susceptible to proteus infection

RM8

A False — it is increasing in frequency

B False — it has no definite benefit over conservative management alone

C False — the typical epidemic variety affects infants and young children, usually presenting with a diarrhoeal prodrome. In these children hypertension, if present, is usually mild whereas older children may have severe hypertension, respiratory problems and central nervous system involvement

D True — activity is low due either to an absence of factors stimulating production or to increased prostacyclin degradation

E False — peritoneal dialysis is the method of choice

RM9

A True

B True

C True — this is due to avid renal retention of sodium in an attempt to increase the intravascular volume

D False — the first sign is tenting of the T waves

E False — it has no effect on the potassium level but stabilises the susceptible myocardial cells

RM10

A True — this may be due to a primary tubular pathology such as Fanconi's syndrome, which is associated with renal tubular acidosis type 1

B False — in orthostatic proteinuria all other tests are usually normal

C False

D True — usually to a low degree

E False — albuminuria suggests glomerular dysfunction

RM11

A False — it accounts for 10–20% of cases of endstage renal failure. In children under 5 years anatomic anomalies predominate. Over 5 years of age acquired lesions such as glomerulonephritis or inherited diseases predominate

B False — the ureters usually emplace in an abnormally lateral position with a shorter intramural section

C True

D True — it is also present in 50% of cases of posterior urethral valves

E False — nearly 80% of cases of grades 1 and 2 resolve spontaneously

RM12

A True

B False — the placenta typically weighs over 40% of the infant's birth weight

C False — proteinuria is usually present at birth

D True — other secondary causes include syphilis, CMV, and toxoplasmosis infections

E True

RM13

A True — most cases present between 2 and 6 years of age

B False — by definition changes are minimal although electron microscopy studies may show changes in epithelial foot processes

C False — the male : female ratio is 2 : 1

D False — the presence of haematuria, hypertension or nephrotic syndrome in an older child should prompt studies for a more sinister cause

E False — they may be raised, and reduced antithrombin 3 levels render patients more vulnerable to venous thromboembolism

RM14

A False

B True — polycystic kidneys or hamartomata are associated with tuberose sclerosis

C False — however, chronic renal failure may occur

D False

E True — enlargement is usually due to hyperplasia. There is an increased incidence of Wilms' tumour, reflecting abnormalities of chromosome 11

RM15

A True

B True

C False
D True — other drugs implicated include cephalosporins, sulphonamides, allopurinol, ranitidine and non-steroidal anti-inflammatory
drugs
E False ?

15: Respiratory Medicine

Answers to this section are to be found
between pages 131 and 134

QUESTIONS

R1 In the management of bronchopulmonary dysplasia (BPD)

A Breathing heliox (a mixture of helium and oxygen) causes a decrease in pulmonary resistance

B The threshold for using ribovarin in RSV bronchiolitis is lower than for patients without BPD

C Digoxin reduces pulmonary vascular resistance

D Total parenteral nutrition (TPN) treatment for four to six weeks is ideal

E Transcutaneous oxygen monitoring overestimates arterial Po_2

R2 Causes of pulmonary hypertension include

A Kyphoscoliosis

B High altitude

C Schistosomiasis

D Right to left shunt

E William's syndrome

R3 Bronchopulmonary dysplasia (BPD)

A Is commoner in male infants

B Prodisposes to rickets

C Is less likely in an individual patient if surfactant is used

D Is associated with nephrocalcinosis

E Is associated with systemic hypertension

R4 Adenovirus pneumonia

A Has seasonal peaks of incidence

B Serotypes 1 and 2 are more virulent than others

C Has unilateral hypertranslucency of the chest as a recognised complication

127

D Preceded by a viral infection predisposes to a more severe adenovirus infection

E Causes obliterative bronchiolitis

R5 In respiratory distress syndrome

A The functional residual capacity is normal

B There is increased dead space

C Expiratory resistance is increased

D The pulmonary artery pressure is increased

E There is contraction of the constrictor muscle of the larynx

R6 The following statements regarding kyphoscoliosis are correct

A Ventilation perfusion mismatch may be found

B Influenza vaccination is indicated

C An altered FEV_1 : FVC ratio can occur

D The more severe type (requiring surgery) is more common in boys

E Cervicothoracic kyphoscoliosis progresses more rapidly

R7 In the treatment of asthma

A Corticosteroids cause reduction in IgE function

B Sodium cromoglycate has a central respiratory stimulatory action

C Theophylline causes enhanced contractility of fatigued respiratory
muscles

D Inhaled steroid treatment may lead to dysphonia

E Beta-2-selective agonists cause enuresis

R8 Causes of persistent stridor include

A *Cri du chat* syndrome

B Subglottic tracheal webs

C Visceral larva migrans

D Kartagener's syndrome (ciliary dyskinesia)

E Lobar emphysema

R9 In meconium aspiration syndrome

A Five to fifteen per cent of term deliveries are affected

B Clinical confusion with persistent pulmonary hypertension may
exist

C The ultimate prognosis is dictated by the degree of respiratory
compromise

D The degree of respiratory compromise may be predicted by measurement of fetal scalp blood pH

E Suction of the subglottic airway should only be carried out after intubation

R10 Indications for sweat testing include

A Pansinusitis

B Rectal prolapse

C Coarctation of the aorta

D Haemoptysis

E Recurrent cystitis

R11 In cystic fibrosis

A The defective gene is located on chromosome 6

B The delta-F508 mutation causes a deletion of a short polypeptide from the gene product

C The delta-F508 mutation causes primarily defective chloride secretion in the sweat duct

D Atrophy of the vas deferens occurs

E The incidence is about 1 in 20 000 live births

R12 Surfactant

A Maturation is faster in a presenting twin

B Synthesis is stimulated by glucocorticoids

C Prevents alveolar collapse

D Function is defective in hypothermic babies

E Administration has decreased the overall incidence of chronic lung disease

R13 The following statements regarding asthma are correct

A The functional residual capacity is increased

B Eosinophilia implies aspergillus superinfection

C Histamine provocation testing is more clinically useful than exercise testing

D In status asthmaticus a normal P_{CO_2} is a reassuring finding

E In status asthmaticus hyperkalaemia is an associated finding

R14 Cystic adenometoid malformation of the lung

A Usually affects one lobe only

B Is characterised histologically by normal lung tissue compressed by cartilagenous cysts

C May be asymptomatic in childhood

D Is more common than lobar emphysema

E Despite surgical resection still renders patients more likely to suffer primary pulmonary neoplasms later in life

R15 In distinguishing viral croup from bacterial epiglottitis

A Croup is characterised by a history of coryzal symptoms

B High fever suggests epiglottitis

C Drooling suggests epiglottitis

D Absence of suprasternal recession suggests croup

E A previous similar episode suggests croup

ANSWERS

R1

A True

B True — this is also true for children with significant congenital heart disease due to their lower cardiopulmonary reserves

C False — cor pulmonale secondary to bronchopulmonary dysplasia may be worsened by digoxin

D False — TPN may be required initially but oral feeds are usually adequate with fewer complications

E False — transcutaneous monitoring usually underestimates Po_2

R2

A True — kyphoscoliosis can cause restrictive lung disease, pulmonary hypertension and hence 'cor pulmonale'

B True — unaccustomed inhalation of air which has a low oxygen tension results in an elevation of the pulmonary artery pressure

C True — in South America and Africa this is the commonest cause of pulmonary hypertension. It is rare below the age of 10 years as emboli of the ova do not reach the lungs until hepatic involvement has produced portal hypertension and collateral channels that bypass the liver

D False — a left to right shunt causes pulmonary hypertension

E False — peripheral pulmonary artery stenosis occurs. The more characteristic lesion is supravalvular aortic stenosis with hypercalcaemia

R3

A True

B False

C True — although surfactant treatment means more children survive who would previously have died and therefore the incidence of BPD appears to be increasing

D True — due to the use of diuretic therapy in treatment

E False — pulmonary hypertension occurs

R4

A True — it is most prevalent in spring and early summer

B False — serotypes 3, 7 and 21 characteristically cause the most severe pneumonias

C True

D True

E True

R5

A False — the functional residual capacity, total lung volumes and compliance are reduced

B True — this is due to absence of gas exchange surfaces in collapsed or absent alveoli

C True — grunting is a physiological attempt at maintaining a positive airway pressure at the end of expiration. The airway closes and resistance to expiration increases

D True — high pulmonary artery pressure falls in normal neonates at birth. Persistence of 'fetal' levels of pressure may make ventilation very difficult

E True

R6

A True

B True — if the kyphoscoliosis causes respiratory compromise

C False — restrictive lung disease causes an equal reduction of both measurements

D False — the female : male ratio in severe scoliosis is 7 : 1

E True

R7

A True — they also have an anti-inflammatory effect and cause increased beta-2 receptor responsiveness

B False — it causes decreased mediator release from mast cells

C True

D True — this is unusual in childhood but may occur. It may be due to a local steroid myopathy of the muscles of phonation

E False

R8

A True

B True

C False — this is a cause of recurrent wheeze
D False — this is a cause of chronic wheeze and cough
E True — this may cause extrinsic compression of a large airway

R9

A False — meconium staining of the liquor occurs in 5–15% of deliveries but aspiration syndrome is much rarer
B True — clinically confusion may occur but the radiological characteristics are quite different, meconium aspiration having areas of atelectasis and air trapping
C False — central nervous system injury from hypoxia determines long-term prognosis
D False
E False — a suction catheter may be passed through the vocal cords before intubation

R10

A True — this is a feature of cystic fibrosis
B True — another feature of cystic fibrosis
C False
D True — also a feature of cystic fibrosis
E False

R11

A False — the gene is on the long arm of chromosome 7
B False — a point mutation at delta-F508 causes deletion of a single phenylalanine residue
C False — chloride absorption is affected
D True — there may be atrophy or absence of the vas deferens and males with cystic fibrosis are almost universally azoospermic
E False — the incidence is approximately 1 in 2000 live births

R12

A True
B True — hence paediatricians' keeness for mothers in preterm labour to be treated with glucocorticoids
C True
D True
E False — since the introduction of surfactant therapy babies that

would previously have died of respiratory distress syndrome have survived

R13

A True

B False — eosinophilia is a common finding in many allergic disorders

C False — exercise testing is more user-friendly and less time-consuming

D False — a normal Pco_2 in a hyperventilating patient is a worrying result and may imply impending respiratory failure

E False — hypokalaemia is more common due to use of aminophylline and beta-agonist therapy

R14

A True — adjacent lobes may be compressed by the abnormal lobe

B False — there is no normal lung tissue in the affected lobe

C True

D False — lobar emphysema is the commonest congenital lung lesion

E True

R15

A True — coryza is usually present for 12–24 h in croup. A short history of cough or stridor is more suggestive of epiglottitis

B True

C True

D False

E True

16: Surgery

*Answers to this section are to be found
between pages 138 and 141*

QUESTIONS

S1 In pyloric stenosis

A There is a higher concordance in monovular twins compared to
binovular twins

B The muscular thickening is confined to the pyloric sphincter

C Hypochloremic alkalosis is found

D The vomitus is bile-stained

E The string sign is seen on contrast study

S2 Diaphragmatic herniae

A That present early in postnatal life have a more favourable
outcome

B Are commonest in the posteromedial part of the diaphragm

C Are associated with pulmonary hypoplasia

D Result from failed closure of pleuroperitoneal canals

E That are associated with a pneumothorax have a worse prognosis

S3 Hirschsprung's disease

A Is more common in premature infants

B Is usually confined to the internal anal sphincter

C Is associated with rectal bleeding

D Is associated with huge stools

E Is diagnosed on rectal biopsy

S4 In inguinal herniae in infants and children

A Conservative management is indicated in the absence of strangu-
lation

B There is a higher incidence on the right side

C The male : female incidence is 10 : 1

D The sac occasionally contains an ovary in females

E Preterm infants are more commonly affected

S5 Intussusception

A Has seasonal peaks in winter and summer
B Is usually ileocolic following surgery
C Is difficult to demonstrate on barium enema if the involved segments are ileoileal
D Is more difficult to diagnose in a child who already has gastroenteritis
E Is more likely to be reduced by barium enema if caused by a polyp or diverticulum

S6 Undescended testes

A Are bilateral in 50% of cases
B Should be surgically fixed at around 5 years of age if detected in infancy
C Occur more commonly in those with anencephaly
D Are associated with infertility irrespective of treatment
E Are more likely to develop malignancy

S7 Oesophagitis

A Due to herpes simplex frequently reveals vesicular lesions on the pharnyx
B Due to candida occurs in the absence of oral candidiasis
C Following ingesting of household cleaning products requires gastric lavage as first-line management
D May cause iron deficiency anaemia
E Is most commonly due to reflux of gastric acid

S8 Osteoid osteoma

A Usually occurs in females
B Is a malignant tumour
C Usually involves the spine and humerus
D Is accompanied by sclerotic changes on X-ray
E Is characterised by severe pain at night

S9 Suspected high anorectal lesions

A Are associated with vertebral anomalies
B Are those lesions that occur above the puborectalis muscle
C Should prompt early radiological investigation
D Result from failure of ascent of the cloaca
E Are associated with genito-urinary abnormalities

S10 Perthes' disease

A Usually affects males

B Has a peak incidence of presentation of 10–12 years

C Is usually bilateral

D Usually has an acute onset

E Is associated with the mucopolysaccharidoses

ANSWERS

S1

A True — it is also more common in males, especially first born and especially if the mother was affected in her infancy

B False — several centimetres of the antrum may show muscular hypertrophy

C True — this is due to the loss of hydrogen and chloride ions. Hypokalaemia is also a feature

D False — bile does not pass back through the hypertrophied pylorus

E True — the string sign is a narrow streak of contrast medium in the stenosed pyloric canal. The stomach may also be enlarged

S2

A False — early presentation is due to severe respiratory embarrassment, commonly with mediastinal shift and compression of the contralateral lung. A nasogastric tube should be on free drainage to decompress the intrathoracic bowel loops. Delayed presentation implies more cardiorespiratory stability

B False — they are usually posterolateral, more often on the left than right

C True — pulmonary arterial muscle hypertrophy may be present in the compressed and hypoplastic ipsilateral lung and pulmonary hypertensive crises are a common problem postoperatively

D True

E True — the ipsilateral lung is usually hypoplastic. Contralateral pneumothorax is poorly tolerated and must be treated promptly

S3

A False — it is more common in term infants with a male : female ratio of 4 : 1

B False — so-called 'ultrashort segment' disease is unusual. Eighty per cent extend to the rectosigmoid junction, 15% to the hepatic flexure and 5% to the ileum

C False — this is usually associated with functional constipation and the passage of hard stools

D False — the stools are usually semiformed or pellet-like. The classic description is of 'ribbon-like' stools

E True — a biopsy to submucosal depth is required. The diagnosis is made in the absence of ganglionic cells within the submucosa. Manometry may also be helpful

S4

A False — all hernias should be treated surgically. Most inguinal hernias are indirect

B True — this may be related to the later descent of the right testis

C True

D True — an ovary may prolapse into a hernia and inspection should be carried out to ensure that it is an ovary and not a testis as may occur in testicular feminisation. If bilateral hernias occur in females and contain 'ovaries' chromosomal analysis may be performed to rule out this condition

E True — it is especially common in previously ventilated preterm children

S5

A False — spring and summer peaks are typical. This is similar to peaks of adenovirus infection

B False — ileoileal intussusception may follow surgery particularly if the small bowel has been handled

C True — a barium enema will demonstrate well both ileocolic and colocolic intussusceptions

D True — abdominal pain and bloody stools may complicate gastro-enteritis

E False — pathological lead points usually fail to reduce with air or contrast enemas and require open reduction

S6

A False — bilateral undescended testes occur in 20–30% of cases. If associated with hypospadias the infant should have its chromosomes checked in case it is a virilised female

B False — spontaneous descent is rare after the age of 1 year and orchidopexy should be performed before the age of 5 years

C True — there is an increased incidence of undescended testis in children with cerebral anomalies

D True — males with undescended testes are less fertile than normal due to testicular atrophy

E True — 0.7% of adult males are cryptorchid. The risk of neoplasm is 30–40% before 50 years of age, 60% being seminomas. Orchidopexy does not eradicate the problem but brings the testis into a position where it may be easier to detect malignancy

S7

A True

B True — candida oesophagitis occurs largely in immunosuppressed patients

C False — these products may be corrosive and emesis or lavage should not be undertaken

D True — this is due to chronic repeated blood loss. Melaena is rare

E True

S8

A False — it is more common in males

B False — it is a benign bone tumour. Treatment is by surgical removal of the tumour

C False — the femur and tibia are the most common sites

D True — the typical finding is a radiolucency with a densely sclerotic ring of bone surrounding it

E True — this may be the presenting feature

S9

A True — the VATER association is Vertebral anomalies, Anorectal atresia, Tracheo oEsophageal fistula and Radial anomalies

B True — clinically high lesions are suggested by vertebral anomalies and poor anal dimple

C False — delayed films at 18–24 h allow swallowed air to reach the anorectal area and the level of obstruction can be diagnosed on lateral films in the prone position with buttocks elevated

D False — high lesions result from failure of descent of the cloaca

E True — faeculent matter may be passed per urethram and cystoscopy and urogenital imaging studies may be necessary

S10

A True — the male : female ratio is 4–5 : 1

B False — the disease presents in the 2–10 year age group with a peak incidence of presentation at 4–6 years

C False — it is bilateral in 10% of cases
D False — the onset is usually insidious over weeks to months
E True — other associations include congenital dislocation of the hip, rickets, and achondroplasia

17: Therapeutics

*Answers to this section are to be found
between pages 145 and 147*

QUESTIONS

TH1 Regarding cytotoxic drugs

A Peripheral neuropathy is a common side effect of vincristine therapy

B L-asparaginase is administered orally

C Platinum-containing drugs cause a more profound thrombocytopenia than other drugs

D Intrathecal vincristine therapy is part of the treatment of acute lymphoblastic leukaemia

E Doxorubicin causes a proximal neuropathy

TH2 Frusemide therapy

A Is associated with an acute increase in lung compliance in the treatment of bronchopulmonary dysplasia

B Increases urinary excretion of chloride

C May lead to hypernatraemia

D Leads to metabolic acidosis

E May lead to neophrolithiasis

TH3 The following drugs should be avoided in porphyria

A Paracetamol

B Salbutamol

C Erythromycin

D Diazepam

E Phenytoin

TH4 Regarding anticonvulsants

A Valproate is the drug of choice in myoclonic seizures

B Carbamazepine doses must be increased slowly

C Phenytoin causes gingival hyperplasia

D Paraldehyde may be given orally

E Lamotrigine is the drug of choice for *petit mal* or simple absence seizures

TH5 Paracetamol

A Has marked anti-inflammatory activity
B Is used in the management of post-immunisation pyrexia
C Is available as an oral, rectal or intravenous preparation
D Toxicity may develop at lower plasma concentrations if a patient is on phenytoin
E Overdose which is fatal is usually due to renal failure

TH6 Penicillin

A Is bacteriostatic
B Has good penetration into the CSF
C Excretion in the renal tubules is enhanced by probenicid
D Given intrathecally may cause fatal encephalopathy
E Is the drug of choice for campylobacter enteritis

TH7 At a cardiac arrest

A Due to ventricular fibrillation the first step is defibrillation at 2 J/kg
B Intubation should be attempted immediately
C Increasing preload may help
D The maximum endotracheal (ET) dose of adrenaline is double the intravenous dose
E The ET dose of lignocaine is double the intravenous dose

TH8 Theophylline

A Is a beta-2 adrenoceptor stimulant
B Is excreted by the kidneys
C Has a reduced half-life when erythromycin is prescribed concurrently
D In overdose causes hyperkalaemia
E May cause supraventricular and ventricular arrhythmias

TH9 The following drug interactions occur

A Metoclopramide accelerates absorption of paracetamol
B Cimetidine enhances metabolism of carbamazepine
C Rifampicin may cause failure of oral contraceptives

D Penicillins increase excretion of methotrexate
E Carbamazepine reduces theophylline levels

TH10 Tricyclic antidepressants

A Are used in the treatment of nocturnal enuresis
B Are contraindicated in patients with diabetes
C Should be used with caution in patients with cardiac disease
D Cause antimuscurinic side effects
E Are useful in the management of night terrors

ANSWERS

TH1

A True

B False — it is administered subcutaneously

C True

D False — intrathecal vincristine is almost universally fatal. Methotrexate for intrathecal use is a different (orange) colour to aid its differentiation from colourless vincristine

E False — its characteristic side effect is cardiotoxicity. Patients on doxorubicin are followed with regular ECHO tests of cardiac function

TH2

A True

B True — it increases urinary excretion of chloride, sodium and potassium, and therefore may lead to hypochloraemia, hyponatraemia and hypokalaemia

C False

D False — it may lead to metabolic alkalosis

E True — chronic diuretic therapy may cause hypercalcuria, renal calcification and nephrolithiasis

TH3

A False

B False

C True

D False

E True

Many drugs induce acute porphyric crises and great care should be taken when prescribing for those known to have porphyria

TH4

A True

B True

C True — it may also cause coarse facies, acne, hirsutism and cerebellar ataxia

D False — it is given by deep intramuscular injection, intravenously or rectally

E False — it is used as adjunctive treatment of partial seizures and secondary generalised tonic–clonic seizures which are not satisfactorily controlled by other drugs. Ethosuxamide and sodium valproate are the drugs of choice for simple absence seizures

TH5
A False — it has no demonstrable anti-inflammatory activity
B True
C False — there is no intravenous preparation
D True — enzyme-inducing drugs, for example carbamazepine, phenobarbitone or rifampicin, may cause toxicity at lower plasma paracetamol concentrations
E False — severe hepatocellular failure is the usual cause of death

TH6
A False — penicillins are bactericidal
B False — penetration into the CSF is poor except when the meninges are inflamed
C False — probenicid blocks the renal tubular excretion of penicillins producing higher and more prolonged plasma concentrations
D True
E False — the recommended antibacterial therapy for campylobacter enteritis is erythromycin or ciprofloxacin

TH7
A True
B False — chin lift and jaw thrust manoeuvres may be adequate to clear the airway
C True — acidosis from poor perfusion may make resuscitation difficult. Volume support may be crucial
D False — the ET dose may be up to ten times that of the intravenous dose
E True
Cardiac arrest in children is usually primarily of a respiratory origin with progressive acidosis. In contrast in adults a primary heart problem is more common and acidosis less common. Airway, Breathing, Circulation is equally important in adults and children

TH8

A False — it is thought to act by inhibition of phosphodiesterase
B False — it is metabolised by the liver
C False — the half-life is increased when prescribed with erythromycin and cimetidine
D False — hypokalaemia is a risk
E True

TH9

A True
B False — it inhibits metabolism of carbamazepine and phenytoin
C True — due to accelerated metabolism there is a reduced contraceptive effect of both the combined and progestogen only oral contraceptive pill. This is important when giving prophylactic rifampicin to contacts of patients with meningococcal meningitis
D False
E True

TH10

A True — they should not be used for longer than a three-week period
B False — contraindications include porphyria, mania, heart block and recent myocardial infarction
C True — side effects include arrhythmias, tachycardia, syncope and postural hypotension
D True — dry mouth, sedation, blurred vision, constipation, nausea and difficulty with micturition all occur
E False

18: Test Paper

Answers to this section are to be found between pages 160 and 176

QUESTIONS

T1 School refusers
A Have poor academic performance
B Are conformist at school
C Display separation anxiety behaviour
D Are reluctant to leave home in the morning
E Continue with neurotic symptoms and social impairment in adulthood in 80% of cases

T2 Causes of elevated maternal serum alpha-fetoprotein (AFP) include
A William's syndrome
B Exomphalos
C Teratoma
D Threatened abortion
E Edwards' syndrome

T3 In the triple X syndrome
A Short stature is the norm
B Premature ovarian failure may occur
C Delayed speech development is a frequent problem
D Coarctation of the aorta is common
E IQ is lower than in controls

T4 Cerebrospinal fluid (CSF) demonstrates the following features
A An elevated glucose level in sarcoidosis
B Low pressure in the presence of a spinal epidural abscess
C A normal glucose level in leptospirosis
D A predominantly lymphocytic leucocytosis in a subdural empyema
E The presence of acid-fast bacilli in tuberculous meningitis

T5 Hirschsprung's disease

A Is commoner in males than females

B Is commonly associated with encopresis

C Presents a more severe clinical picture in breast fed babies

D Is suggested by the passage of pellet stools

E Is characterised by an aganglionic segment which extends from the anus to the hepatic flexure

T6 Unconjugated hyperbilirubinaemia occurs in

A Hypothyroidism

B Budd–Chiari syndrome

C Pyruvate kinase deficiency

D Spherocytosis

E Prolonged intravenous nutrition

T7 In Kawasaki's disease

A Forty per cent of patients develop coronary artery aneurysms

B There is an association with thrombocytopenia

C Constipation is characteristic

D Geographic tongue is common

E Skin peeling off on the extremities is an early sign

T8 In Prader–Willi syndrome

A There is hypertonia

B The penis is small

C Weight is usually below the third centile

D Hands and feet are small

E The hair is often blonde

T9 Arthritis occurs in

A Lyme disease

B Haemolytic uraemic syndrome

C Sickle cell disease

D Hodgkin's disease

E Addison's disease

T10 Talipes equinovarus

A Is more common in males

B Is associated with polyhydramnios

C Is commonly bilateral
D Is characterised by abnormal plantar flexion
E Requires early splinting

T11 Rheumatic fever
A Is associated with painful arthritis
B Is associated with a short P–R interval
C Does not recur
D Is frequently the result of streptococcal skin infections
E Has a peak incidence between 1 and 3 years

T12 With regard to the eye
A Most newborn infants are mildly hypermetropic
B There is a high prevalence of astigmatism in infancy
C The peripheral retina is poorly developed at birth
D The defect in ocular coloboma is usually in the 1 or 2 o'clock position
E Persistent divergent squint is usually of no significance

T13 Causes of inappropriate ADH secretion include
A Guillain–Barré syndrome
B Cystic fibrosis
C Perinatal asphyxia
D Erythromycin therapy
E Pyridoxine deficiency

T14 In Pendred's syndrome (congenital hypothyroidism with deafness)
A There is a deficiency in iodide peroxidase
B Inheritance is usually autosomal dominant
C Most affected persons are clinically euthyroid
D Hearing loss is usually more pronounced in the lower frequencies
E IQ is usually 50–70

T15 The following statements regarding trace elements and minerals are correct
A Chloride may become deficient following excessive sweating
B Manganese is found in high concentration in meat
C Zinc deficiency causes hypogonadism

D More than 70% of ingested calcium is excreted in the urine
E Molybdenum excess causes tetany

T16 With regard to poisoning
A Iron ingestion is the commonest form in childhood
B Haemodialysis is used in the management of lithium poisoning
C Nystagmus occurs in alcohol intoxication
D Activated charcoal enhances the elimination of theophylline
E Liver damage is maximal 24–48 h following paracetamol ingestion

T17 Hyperammonaemia in the newborn
A May be transient and mild
B Is suggested by hepatomegaly and coma
C That is associated with acidosis suggests ornithine transcarbamylase deficiency
D Requires a high calorie, low protein intake
E May be treated with sodium benzoate

T18 Kwashiokor is characterised by
A Immune deficiency
B Fatty infiltration of the liver
C Normal glucose tolerance
D Decreased glomerular filtration rate
E Decreased alkaline phosphatase

T19 A term infant
A Requires a larger fluid intake per unit weight than an adult
B Retains 20% of ingested water
C Loses 50% of ingested fluid insensibly
D Has a calorie requirement of 200–250 kcal/kg/day
E Prefers faces rather than geometric shapes to look at

T20 Night terrors
A Are recalled on morning waking
B Are related to transition from stage 1 to stage 2 sleep
C Are characterised by unresponsiveness to parents' comforting manoeuvres
D Are associated with sleepwalking
E Are more common in girls

T21 Anaphylaxis

A Is associated with stridor

B Is dose-dependent

C Is more severe for injected substances

D Should be treated with beta-adrenergic blockade

E Is IgE mediated

T22 The following are notifiable infectious diseases

A Tetanus

B Acute meningitis

C Food poisoning

D Whooping cough

E Bronchiolitis

T23 Recognised complications of infectious mononucleosis include

A Agranulocytosis

B Pneumonitis

C Exophthalmos

D Thrombocytosis

E Pericarditis

T24 The following statements regarding mumps are correct

A Infection is spread by droplet infection

B The incubation period is 7–10 days

C The virus can be isolated from urine

D Epididymo-orchitis is commoner in young boys

E The submandibular gland alone is involved in 50% of cases

T25 In ventricular septal defects (VSDs)

A Multiple defects are more common than single defects

B The majority of defects involve the membranous septum

C The murmur radiates to the back

D The shunt is reversed in Eisenmenger syndrome

E Changes in the lungs are reversible if the defect is surgically corrected before the age of 10 years

T26 In egg allergy

A Cooked egg white is more allergenic than raw egg white

B Onset of symptoms is usually immediate

C Skin prick test positivity may persist for years after clinical resolution
D Children should avoid marshmallows
E MMR vaccine is contraindicated

T27 Congential dislocation of the hip
A Is more common in males
B Affects both hips in 20% of cases
C Has a higher incidence following breech delivery
D Has a recurrence risk of less than 10% in future pregnancies
E Is best confirmed by X-ray in the neonatal period

T28 The umbilical vein
A Becomes the umbilical ligament when it atrophies
B Should be used for dilutional exchange transfusion
C Is commonly double
D May be anatomically patent for two weeks
E Is usually in spasm after ligation of the cord

T29 There are effects on the fetus from maternal
A Diabetes mellitus
B Cocaine use
C Sickle cell trait
D Systemic lupus erythematosus (SLE)
E Paracetamol

T30 Anorexia nervosa
A Occurs in all social classes
B Is more common than bulimia nervosa
C Is associated with passage of loose stools
D Has a mortality rate of 0.5%
E Is associated with low levels of growth hormone

T31 Infantile hypertrophic pyloric stenosis
A Is five times more common in males
B Should be treated by emergency pyloromyotomy
C Is associated with conjugated hyperbilirubinaemia
D Is suggested by an ultrasound measurement of pyloric length of greater than or equal to 14 mm
E Is characterised by a hungry baby

T32 Hypoplastic left heart syndrome
A Usually presents in low birthweight infants
B Is associated with oliguria
C Shows right axis deviation on electrocardiogram
D Is the commonest cause of heart failure in the first few days of life
E May be difficult to distinguish from septicaemia

T33 Intraventricular haemorrhage
A Occurs in the first 24 h in 60% of cases
B May cause decreased CSF glucose concentrations
C Results from damage to the middle cerebral artery
D Occurs in 60–70% of babies less than 750 g
E Is associated with decreased cerebral blood flow

T34 Short stature is found in
A Homocystinuria
B Down's syndrome
C Marfan's syndrome
D Hypothyroidism
E Klinefelter's syndrome

T35 Inactivated vaccines include
A Oral polio
B Diphtheria
C Tetanus
D Yellow fever
E Influenza

T36 In haemolytic uraemic syndrome
A Coagulation abnormalities are common
B Macroscopic haematuria occurs
C The presence of a diarrhoeal prodrome is a favourable feature
D Older children have a worse prognosis
E Renal biopsy is necessary to confirm diagnosis

T37 Drowning
A Is the commonest cause of accidental death in children
B Most commonly occurs in seawater
C May be complicated by cervical spine injury

D Should prompt urgent measurement of the axillary temperature

E May require gastric lavage

T38 Coeliac disease

A Presents in 20% of first-degree relatives of proven cases

B May present as constipation

C Is excluded by the absence of IgA anti-gliadin antibodies on serological testing

D Has a characteristic intraepithelial eosinophilia on intestinal mucosal biopsy

E Is commonest in Africans

T39 Classical phenylketonuria (PKU)

A Is commonly associated with evidence of hypertonia on physical examination

B Is associated with dental enamel hypoplasia

C May be difficult to diagnose on serum phenylalanine levels alone in the newborn

D Is caused by a deficiency of phenylalanine hydroxylase

E Has serum phenylalanine levels of 700 μmol/l in an untreated neonate

T40 In infective endocarditis

A Cutaneous signs are common

B Bacteraemia is intermittent

C A predisposing risk factor is rarely found

D Leucocytosis is a common finding

E Haematuria is embolically mediated

T41 In atopic dermatitis

A Serum IgE is raised in 80% of patients

B The condition usually begins on the scalp

C Extensor surface disease usually precedes flexural disease

D Bath oil should be put in the water before the child enters the bath

E Infected lesions should be treated with topical antibiotics

T42 The following are major criteria for the diagnosis of rheumatic fever

A Arthralgia

B Chorea
C Fever
D Subcutaneous nodules
E Prolonged P–R interval on ECG

T43 Associations of hydrops fetalis include
A Biliary atresia
B Maternal asthma
C Parvovirus infection
D Turner's syndrome
E Umbilical vein thrombosis

T44 In salicylate poisoning
A Respiratory alkalosis is a significant early feature
B Phenistix go red-brown in colour on testing the urine
C An emetic is only effective up to 4 h post-ingestion
D Hyperkalaemia may be marked
E Tinnitus implies ingestion of significant amounts of salicylate

T45 Hypocalcaemia
A In a neonate may be the result of maternal hyperparathyroidism
B That is associated with a low phosphate and high alkaline phosphatase is suggestive of rickets
C With a high phosphate and high parathyroid hormone occurs in hypoparathyroidism
D Is more common than hypercalcaemia in children
E Occurs in Addison's disease

T46 In the tetralogy of Fallot
A The systolic murmur becomes louder during the hypercyanotic attack
B The second heart sound is single
C Anaemia is a complication
D A Blalock–Taussig shunt anastomoses the ascending aorta to the right pulmonary artery
E The pulmonary vascular markings may be asymmetrical

T47 In rickets
A Craniotabes is a late sign

B There is characteristic cupping of the distal ends of the radius and ulna

C Urinary cyclic AMP is reduced

D There may be normal calcium levels

E Early closure of the fontanelle occurs

T48 Characteristics of Henoch–Schoenlein purpura include

A A low platelet count

B Skin lesions which initially blanch on pressure

C Reduced complement levels

D Prolonged thromboplastin time

E Elevated rheumatoid factor levels

T49 Lead poisoning

A Is associated with pica

B Causes defective myoglobin synthesis

C May cause Fanconi's syndrome

D May cause cerebral oedema in young children

E Should be treated with desferrioxamine

T50 In insulin-dependent diabetes mellitus

A The concordance rate for monozygotic twins is 90%

B Islet cell antibodies are found in 90% of newly diagnosed patients

C C peptide may be in serum for several years

D The daily dose of insulin should be reduced during intercurrent illness

E Islet delta cell function is decreased

T51 In Hunter's syndrome (mucopolysaccharidosis 2)

A The skeletal defects are more severe than in Hurler's syndrome (mucopolysaccharidosis 1S)

B Corneal clouding is absent

C There is commonly associated hearing loss

D Inheritance is as an autosomal recessive trait

E Enzyme levels determine the severity of the disease

T52 Phaeochromocytomas

A Are associated with neurofibromatosis

B Are malignant in 50% of cases

C Develop from chromaffin cells

D Cause hypertension in childhood which is usually paroxysmal

E Are associated with polydypsia and polyuria

T53 Hypoglycaemia occurs in

A Salicylate overdose

B Hypothermia

C Beckwith–Wiedemann syndrome

D Fulminant hepatitis

E Birth asphyxia

T54 An overdose of tricyclic drugs is associated with

A Hypertension

B Pin-point pupils

C Auditory hallucinations

D Hyporeflexia

E Arrhythmias

T55 In typhoid fever

A Ulceration of Peyer's patches occurs

B Spread may be by infected ice-cream

C Glomerulonephritis may be due to immune complex disease

D Hypernatraemia is common

E *Salmonella typhi* may be cultured from rose spots

T56 In Pierre Robin syndrome

A Cleft lip is a frequent finding

B The tongue is normal in size

C Babies should be nursed in a supine position

D A normal facial appearance can develop without corrective surgery

E Congenital glaucoma occurs

T57 In meningococcal septicaemia

A The coexistence of meningitic signs worsens the prognosis

B Patients in whom the diagnosis is suspected should not be treated until blood cultures are obtained

C Blood cultures are usually positive

D Corticosteroid therapy is beneficial

E The causative organism is a Gram-positive diplococcus

T58 Ventricular septal defects are characterised by

A Ejection systolic murmurs

B Pulmonary plethora

C Cyanosis

D Typical ECHO findings in the first 4 h of life

E A loud pulmonary 2nd sound

T59 Alpha-1 antitrypsin deficiency

A Causes neonatal cholestasis

B Is characterised by the Pi MM genotype in homozygotes

C Causes bronchiectasis in the first decade

D Requires liver biopsy for definitive diagnosis

E Is more common in Northern Europeans

T60 In systemic onset juvenile chronic arthritis

A Iridocyclitis is common

B Fever is low grade

C Joint involvement may be delayed

D HLA B27 positivity is common

E The presentation may mimic malignant disease

ANSWERS

T1

A False — most have good academic attainment

B True — they may be conformist at school but oppositional at home

C True — this is often also evident in the mother and this may exacerbate the child's anxiety

D True — in contrast to the truant who leaves home but never arrives at school

E False — Two-thirds return to school regularly and only one-third achieve erratic attendance. One-third continue with neurotic symptoms and social impairment

T2

A False

B True — alpha-fetoprotein is produced by the yolk sac and structures that are derived from the yolk sac. When such structures are exposed to the amniotic fluid by developmental abnormalities the maternal levels of AFP rise. Such abnormalities include gastroschisis, myelomeningocele, anencephaly, Turner's syndrome and haemangioma of the placenta or cord

C True

D True — other causes include multiple pregnancy and intrauterine death

E False

T3

A False — most of these females are taller than average

B True — gonadal function is usually normal but premature ovarian failure may occur

C True — about 50% of affected girls have delayed speech development

D False — apart from being taller most are physically normal

E True

T4

A False — the glucose level is usually normal

B True

C True

D False — polymorphs predominate
E True

T5

A True — four males are affected to every one female
B False — in the older child constipation and abdominal distension occur. In the rarer form of ultrashort-segment Hirschsprung's disease, encopresis may occur
C False — bottle fed babies manifest a more severe clinical picture
D True — stools may be pellet-like, ribbon-like or have a fluid consistency. Large stools as found in functional constipation are rare
E False — in 80% the aganglionic segment is limited to the rectosigmoid region

T6

A True
B False — this causes hepatic vein thrombosis
C True — this is a rare cause of haemolysis
D True — this causes haemolysis
E False — this causes conjugated hyperbilirubinaemia

T7

A True — the aneurysms are secondary to vasculitis of the coronary arteries and are usually evident in the first few weeks of the illness. Repeated ECHO studies are indicated
B False — thrombocythaemia occurs
C False — diarrhoea occurs
D False — a strawberry tongue occurs
E False — this generally occurs during the 2nd to 3rd week of the illness
The criteria for diagnosing Kawasaki's disease are fever for more than five days (usually a high fever) and four of the following: conjunctivitis; oral mucocutaneous changes; typical rash; peripheral oedema, peeling or erythema; or cervical adenopathy

T8

A False — hypotonia is a feature of this syndrome, and is often severe in early infancy

B True — the penis is small and there is cryptorchidism
C False — obesity is a feature of the Prader–Willi syndrome
D True
E True — there is usually fair sensitive skin

T9

A True
B False
C True
D True
E False

T10

A True — the male : female ratio is 2 : 1
B False — positional talipes is associated with uterine compression and with oligohydramnios
C True — in 50% of cases
D True — abnormal plantar flexion does not occur in simple positional talipes
E True — treatment should be started in the first week of life. Severe forms may require surgery before one year of age. Positional talipes usually only requires passive manipulation

T11

A True
B False — there may be a long P–R interval (first degree heart block)
C False — it may recur
D False — group A streptococcal impetigo does not usually cause rheumatic fever. Streptococcal throat infections are a more common precedent
E False — peak incidence is 5–15 years

T12

A True
B True
C False — the peripheral retina is relatively well developed but the macular region is immature
D False — the tissue defect is usually in the 6 or 7 o'clock position inferiorly

E False — this is a common condition in the first two months of life but persistent extropia is rare and occurs in children with severe neurological damage

T13

A True

B True

C True

D False — it occurs with the use of vincristine, vinblastine and tetracycline

E False — this causes convulsions in infants, peripheral neuritis, dermatitis and anaemia

T14

A False — the biochemical defect is not known

B False — it is inherited in an autosomal recessive fashion

C True

D False — it is more pronounced at higher frequencies

E False — IQ is normal

T15

A True — also following prolonged vomiting. Patients with cystic fibrosis may need to increase their salt intake in hot weather

B False — it is found in cereals, nuts and green leafy vegetables

C True — zinc deficiency also causes dwarfism, hepatosplenomegaly, hyperpigmentation and acrodermatitis enteropathica

D False — it is 70% excreted in the faeces

E False — the effects of excess molybdenum are unknown

T16

A True

B True

C True

D True

E False — it is more common 3–4 days after ingestion and should be sought by regular testing of coagulation and other liver function tests

T17

A True — the ammonia level is rarely above 150 μmol/l

B True

C False — this disorder of the urea cycle does not cause acidosis but does cause high levels of urinary orotic acid

D True — protein intake should be kept to a minimum level that provides adequate amounts of essential amino acids

E True — this allows excretion of ammonia in the form of hippurate

T18

A True — secondary immunodeficiency is one of the most constant and serious complications

B True

C False — glucose tolerance curves may be similar to those of a diabetic

D True

E True

T19

A True — an infant needs approximately 150 ml/kg/day as compared to 75–80 ml/kg/day for an adult

B False — the normal retention of water is 0.5–3%

C True

D False — the daily requirement is 80–120 kcal/kg/day until 1 year of age

E True

T20

A False — there is total amnesia the following morning

B False — they occur during stage 3 or 4 of slow-wave sleep

C True — the children are unaware of their parents or their surroundings

D True — about a third of children with night terrors sleepwalk

E False — they are most common in 5–7-year-old boys

T21

A True — acute upper airway obstruction can be caused by angioedema. This may present as stridor. Wheeze due to bronchospasm may also occur

B False — anaphylaxis is immune-mediated and is usually due to IgE-mediated massive mast cell degranulation. This is independent of the dose of allergen

C True

D False — adrenaline subcutaneously is the treatment of choice 1/1000 0.01 mg/kg. Airway support and fluid control are vital. Remember Airway, Breathing, Circulation

E True — occasional anaphylactoid reactions occur on first exposure possibly due to unwitting previous exposure or direct action of the allergen on basophils and mast cells

T22

A True

B True

C True

D True

E False

T23

A True — other complications include meningitis, encephalitis, cranial nerve palsies, polyneuritis, arthritis, respiratory obstruction, agammaglobulinaemia, haemolytic anaemia, splenic rupture, pericarditis and myocarditis

B True

C False

D False — thrombocytopenia may occur

E True

T24

A True

B False — the incubation period is 16–18 days

C True — in about 70% of cases the virus can be isolated from the urine in the first few days of the illness. It can also be isolated from the saliva and CSF

D False — epididymo-orchitis is rare before puberty

E False — the parotid glands are usually involved but in 10% of cases both the submandibular and parotid glands are affected

T25

A False — the defect is usually single

B True

C False

D True — there is a right to left shunt due to pulmonary hypertension

E False — changes are reversible if surgery is carried out before 12 months of age, although in Down's syndrome irreversible changes may occur at an earlier age

T26

A False — cooking reduces allergenicity by 70%

B True — it may happen almost on contact with the oral mucosa. The lips swell and facial flushing typically occurs; laryngeal oedema and stridor may also occur. Delayed reactions include vomiting and a worsening of eczema 2–3 days later

C True — most children allergic to eggs present at around six months of age but are able to tolerate eggs by 3–4 years

D True — the child should avoid Turkish delight and any loose sweets whose ingredients may be uncertain

E False — the vaccine is no longer obtained from chick embryo cultures but from chick embryo fibroblasts which do not contain traces of the typical egg antigens. However reactions have occurred and it may be best to immunise these children in hospital if the allergic reaction to egg is severe

T27

A False — it is more common in girls

B True — the left alone is involved in 60%, the right in 20% and both in 20%

C True

D True

E False — ultrasound is more useful and has no radiation risk

T28

A False — the umbilical vein atrophies to the ligamentum teres

B False — dilutional exchange transfusions are carried out to treat symptomatic polycythaemia which causes a hyperviscosity syndrome. Central arteries and veins should not be used for this procedure

C False — the umbilical vein is usually single

D True — it is possible to catheterise the umbilical vein up to cord separation but it is not desirable because of reasons of sepsis. The umbilical vein closes functionally at the time of cord ligation

E False — the umbilical vein is usually patulous and bleeds easily. The umbilical arteries however are usually in spasm

T29

A True — macrosomia occurs and there is an increased incidence of congenital heart disease

B True — this may cause growth retardation, prematurity, placental abruption and intrauterine cerebral thrombosis

C False — haemoglobin F is resistant to sickling

D True — it may cause congenital heart block

E False — paracetamol is considered safe for use in pregnancy

T30

A True — the incidence is 1% of 16–18-year-old females. It occurs in all social classes.

B False

C False — constipation is a common problem

D False — the mortality rate is about 5%, death occurring mainly from hypothermia, hypoglycaemia and secondary infection

E False — growth hormone levels are high

T31

A True — there is a familial incidence of 15%

B False — this should be done after correction of metabolic abnormalities

C False — it causes an unconjugated hyperbilirubinaemia

D True

E True — this is in contrast to babies who vomit because of overfeeding or have urinary tract infections

T32

A False — the babies usually appear normal at birth

B True — due to low renal blood flow

C True — right axis deviation is a normal finding in neonates

D True

E True — on deterioration the baby may appear pale, collapsed and pulseless

T33

A True — 90% have occurred in the first 72 h
B True — the glucose level is often low due to the high polymorpho-nuclear response
C False — it is due to damage to the capillaries of the germinal matrix
D True — the grade of haemorrhage varies and there may be no long-term sequelae
E True — acidosis and hypothermia may also predispose to IVH

T34

A False — tall stature occurs in this condition
B True
C False — these children may be tall
D True
E False — short stature is not a feature

T35

A False — it is a live virus. Infants in a neonatal unit should not receive oral polio vaccine until discharge
B True
C True
D False — it is a live vaccine
E True

T36

A False — coagulation abnormalities are rarely found
B False — haematuria is usually microscopic
C True — other favourable features include young age and presentation during epidemics
D True
E False — the clinical picture is usually typical and thrombocytopenia precludes biopsy

T37

A False — road traffic accidents and burns are more common causes of fatality. Drowning kills 0.7/100 000 children (less than 15 years of age) per year. The highest incidence is found in boys less than 5 years (3.6/100 000)

B False — most drownings are in private and public swimming pools, ponds and inland waterways

C True — witness accounts of diving should be urgently sought and the cervical spine protected during resuscitation and transfer

D False — a rectal measurement is mandatory. Cooling may have preserved vital organ function and resuscitation should be continued until rewarming to 37°C has been achieved and there is still no sign of life

E True — swallowed debris should be removed after airway protection. Gastric lavage with warm fluids may help rewarming

T38

A False — it presents overtly in 2% of first-degree relatives although 10% will have asymptomatic subtotal villous atrophy on biopsy

B True

C False — jejunal biopsy is the gold standard for diagnosis

D False — the infiltrate is characteristically lymphocytic

E False — it has a higher incidence in Irish, Scots and Scandinavians

T39

A True

B True

C True — normal babies may have increased serum phenylalanine levels for several days. Definitive testing must be undertaken after finding a raised level in a baby established on feeds for 3–5 days

D True — it is inherited in an autosomal recessive manner

E True — the acceptable upper limit for babies up to three months is a serum phenylalanine level of 180 μmol/l

T40

A False — they are rare, late signs of vasculitis and include splinter haemorrhages, tender Osler's nodes in the finger pulps, and painless Janeway lesions on the palms

B False — patients with endocarditis are nearly always bacteraemic

C False — 30% of patients have a predisposing condition such as congenital or rheumatic heart disease

D True — the ESR and CRP may also be elevated

E False — it is an immune complex glomerulonephritis

T41

A True

B False — the earliest lesions are usually on the cheeks with later extension to the face, neck, hands and extensor surfaces

C True

D False — bath oil should be added after the child has soaked in the bath as its purpose is to seal water into the skin

E False — these are of little benefit and may lead to sensitisation. Systemic antibiotics should be used

T42

A False — major criteria are carditis, polyarthritis, erythema marginatum, chorea and subcutaneous nodules

B True

C False — minor criteria include fever, arthralgia, previous rheumatic fever, elevated acute phase reactants (ESR, CRP) and prolonged P–R interval on an electrocardiogram

D True

E False

T43

A True — other hepatic disorders include congenital hepatitis, cirrhosis and vascular tumours

B False — maternal conditions associated with hydrops fetalis include diabetes mellitus, toxaemia and anaemia

C True — other intrauterine infections include rubella, syphilis, toxoplasmosis, herpes simplex type 1 and cytomegalovirus

D True — other chromosomal disorders include trisomies 13, 18 and 21

E True — other placental and cord conditions include chorioangioma, chorionic vein thrombosis and placental insufficiency

T44

A True — hyperventilation is a feature. The development of metabolic acidosis implies significant ingestion or the ingestion of other agents along with the salicylates

B True

C False — salicylates delay gastric emptying and delayed emesis may be indicated

D False — the respiratory alkalosis causes urinary bicarbonate and potassium losses

E True

T45

A True — parathyroid hormone can cross the placenta and cause neonatal hypoparathyroidism characterised by a low calcium and high phosphate level

B True

C False — this would suggest secondary hyperparathyroidism as occurs in chronic renal failure

D True

E False

T46

A False — the blue spells are associated with reduction of pulmonary blood flow and increased right to left shunting

B True — due to pulmonary stenosis

C False — polycythaemia due to chronic hypoxia renders them susceptible to cerebrovascular thrombosis

D False — it anastomoses a subclavian artery to the ipsilateral pulmonary artery either directly or using a teflon graft

E True — asymmetry may be due to the presence of collateral bronchial arteries

T47

A False — this is an early sign of rickets, due to thinning of the outer table of the skull. A ping-pong ball sensation is felt on pressing firmly over the occiput or parietal bones

B True

C False — it is increased

D True — calcium may be normal or low. Serum phosphate is low and serum alkaline phosphatase is elevated

E False — the anterior fontanelle is larger than normal and its closure may be delayed beyond 2 years of age

T48

A False — the platelet count is normal
B True — the lesions initially blanch but lose this feature after becoming petechial or purpuric
C False — serum complement levels are normal or elevated
D False — coagulation studies are normal
E False — neither rheumatoid factor nor anti-nuclear antibody (ANA) are present

T49

A True
B False — sideroblastic anaemia is characteristic. A blue line may be seen on the gums and abdominal pain of a colicky nature occurs
C True
D True — although the classical signs of increased intracranial pressure may not be found
E False — EDTA (given intramuscularly) is used as chelation therapy

T50

A False — the concordance rate is only 30–50%. The peak ages of diagnosis of diabetes are 5–7 years and around puberty
B True — a lymphocytic infiltrate may be seen around the pancreatic islets, possibly reflecting a virally induced or autoimmune destruction of the beta cells that produce insulin
C True — many patients, especially soon after diagnosis, demonstrate detectable but inadequate insulin secretion
D False — with the physiological stress of illness and surgery the usual dose of insulin may be inadequate to counteract the stress hormones of glucagon, cortisol and adrenaline, and the dose may need to be increased
E False — insulin is secreted by beta cells in the islets of Langerhans

T51

A False — it is milder than Hurler's syndrome with respect to skeletal and mental defects
B True
C True

D False — it is the only X-linked disorder among the mucopolysaccharidoses

E False — there is no biochemical or enzymatic difference between the severe form of the disease (type A) and the milder form (type B)

T52

A True — they are usually sporadic but may be familial or part of MEN (multiple endocrine adenopathies) types 1 and 2 or associated with neurofibromatosis

B False — 5–10% are malignant

C True — they can arise from the adrenal medulla or the sympathetic chain in the neck, abdomen or mediastinum

D False — in childhood the hypertension is usually sustained and headaches, sweating and vomiting occur

E True — other features include visual disturbances, abdominal pain and convulsions

T53

A True — it also occurs following alcohol ingestion

B True — there is decreased glucose production following birth asphyxia, sepsis, starvation and hypotonia

C True — hyperinsulinism also occurs in polycythaemia and in infants of diabetic mothers

D True — it also occurs in Reye's syndrome and various inborn errors of metabolism

E True

T54

A False — hypotension occurs

B False — dilated pupils occur

C True — visual hallucinations also occur

D False — hyperreflexia is more common

E True — some will respond to correction of hypoxia and acidosis; the use of antiarrhythmic drugs is best avoided

T55

A True — bacilli are taken up by macrophages in Peyer's patches and an inflammatory reaction results in swelling, necrosis and ulceration

B True — in developed countries spread is usually caused by con-
tamination of food by a carrier. Outbreaks occur from infected milk
and ice-cream. *Salmonella typhi* survives freezing and drying. In
developing countries spread may be via flies, insects or a contaminated water source

C True

D False — hyponatraemia is common

E True

T56

A False — there is no cleft lip. The palate is high-arched or may show
a postalveolar cleft

B True — the tongue is poorly anchored and is displaced downwards
and backwards (glossoptosis)

C False — respiratory distress is aggravated by nursing in the supine
position or by feeding. Nursing should be in the prone position
with the chest and shoulders supported, allowing the tongue to fall
forwards

D True — good jaw growth may occur so that a normal profile is
attained at 4–6 years

E True — other ocular manifestations include strabismus and retinal
detachment

T57

A False — the absence of meningeal irritation imparts a worse
prognosis. Authorities differ regarding the necessity of lumbar
puncture in the presence of obvious septicaemia and vasculitic
skin lesions. Lumbar puncture may cause seeding of the meningo-
coccus into the cerebrospinal fluid

B False — the high mortality (up to 25–30%) demands that treatment is started as early as possible. Unproven penicillin allergy
is not a contraindication to benzylpenicillin given i.v. or i.m.
Family doctors are advised to carry benzylpenicillin for such an
eventuality

C True — blood cultures taken as soon as possible may be positive
despite pretreatment. A throat swab is particularly useful in
diagnosing meningococcal carriage or infection in pretreated cases.
The benefits of latex agglutination testing are unproven

D False — steroids are not of proven benefit in Gram-negative endo-
toxic shock.

E False — *Neisseria meningitidis* is a Gram-negative diplococcus

T58

A False — the murmur is classically pansystolic. Occasionally small
muscular VSDs close in late systole so the typical pansystolic
murmur is replaced by a mid-systolic murmur

B True — VSDs with large left to right shunts cause increased
pulmonary blood flow with 3 : 1 shunts or greater

C False — cyanosis is not a characteristic of VSDs unless right to left
shunting occurs during crying, or Eisenmenger complex develops
in an untreated large VSD

D False — blood flow across the defect may be minimal while the left
ventricle adapts to postnatal life. Defects may not be visible and the
typical colour Doppler appearances of left to right shunting may be
absent

E True — large left to right shunts may cause pulmonary hypertension

T59

A True — in cases of prolonged jaundice cholestasis must be ruled
out to ensure the absence of, among other causes, alpha-1
antitrypsin deficiency and biliary atresia

B False — the PiZZ genotype is associated with severe clinical manifestations. PiMM is the normal genotype

C False — respiratory manifestations are rare in childhood. Basal
panacinar emphysema may develop in adulthood, particularly in
cigarette smokers

D True — inclusion bodies in hepatocytes stain PAS positive and
reflect hepatic inability to secrete alpha-1 antitrypsin

E False

T60

A False — iridocyclitis is a feature of pauciarticular juvenile chronic
arthritis

B False — the fever is usually dramatic with huge peaks and rapid
resolution. The typical rash is classically evanescent, coming and
going very quickly

C True — it may be delayed for several months or even years

D False — HLA B27 is associated with pauciarticular juvenile chronic arthritis (type 2). These patients are usually 8–11-year-old boys with large joint arthritis. Ankylosing spondylitis is associated

E True — systemic onset juvenile chronic arthritis may present with hepatomegaly and lymphadenopathy. Routine microscopy of biopsies may not be helpful

Bibliography

Bacon, C.J. & Lamb, W.H. *Paediatric Emergencies: Diagnosis and Management*, 2nd edn, 1989. Heinemann, Oxford.

Behrman, R.E. (ed.) *Nelson Textbook of Paediatrics*, 14th edn, 1992. W.B. Saunders, Philadelphia.

Brett, E.M. *Paediatric Neurology*, 2nd edn, 1991. Churchill Livingstone, Edinburgh.

British National Formulary, 27th edn, 1994. British Medical Association and Royal Pharmaceutical Society of Great Britain, London.

Campbell, A.G.M. & McIntosh, N. (eds) *Forfar and Arneil Textbook of Paediatrics*, 4th edn, 1992. Churchill Livingstone, Edinburgh.

Guyton, A.C. *Guyton Textbook of Medical Physiology*, 8th edn, 1990. W.B. Saunders, Philadelphia.

Harvey, D. & Kovar, I. *Child Health, a Textbook for the DCH*, 2nd edn, 1991. Churchill Livingstone, Edinburgh.

Her Majesty's Stationery Office. *Immunisation against Infectious Disease*, 2nd edn, 1992. HMSO, London.

Jordan, S.C. & Scott, O. *Heart Disease in Paediatrics*, 3rd edn, 1989. Butterworths, London.

Kingston, H.M. *ABC of Clinical Genetics*, 2nd edn, 1994. British Medical Association, London.

Markowitz, M. (ed.) *Smith's Recognisable Patterns of Human Malformation, Genetic, Embryologic and Clinical Manifestations*, 4th edn, 1992. W.B. Saunders & Co., Philadelphia.

Polnay, L. & Hull, D. *Community Paediatrics*, 1990. Churchill Livingstone, Edinburgh.

Roberton, N.R.C. *Textbook of Neonatalogy*, 2nd edn, 1992. Churchill Livingstone, Edinburgh.

Roitt, I. *Essential Immunology*, 8th edn, 1994. Blackwell Scientific Publications, Oxford.

Rudd, P. & Nicholl, A. (eds) *British Paediatric Association Manual on Infections and Immunizations in Children*, 2nd edn, 1991. Oxford University Press, Oxford.

Strasburger, V.C. & Brown, R.T. *Adolescent Medicine, a Practical Guide*, 1991. Little, Brown & Co., Boston.

Index

Page numbers in **bold** print refer to questions; page numbers inside parentheses refer to their corresponding answers.